STRUCTURAL FITNESS

STRUCTURAL

The essential guide to

John L. Stirk

FITNESS

better body mechanics

Illustrations by Beryl Sanders

ELM TREE BOOKS

For Lolly and Sarah

ELM TREE BOOKS

Published by the Penguin Group
27 Wrights Lane, London W8 5TZ, England
Viking Penguin Inc., 40 West 23rd Street, New York, New York 10010, U.S.A.
Penguin Books Australia Ltd, Ringwood, Victoria, Australia
Penguin Books Canada Ltd, 2801 John Street, Markham, Ontario, Canada L3R 1B4
Penguin Books (N.Z.) Ltd, 182–190 Wairau Road, Auckland 10, New Zealand

Penguin Books Ltd, Registered Offices: Harmondsworth, Middlesex, England

First published in Great Britain 1988 by
Elm Tree Books/Hamish Hamilton Ltd

British Library Cataloguing in Publication Data
Stirk, John
Structural fitness.
1. Exercise 2. Physical fitness
I. Title
613.7'1 RA781

ISBN 0-241-12432-8
ISBN 0-241-12431-X Pbk

Printed and bound in Great Britain by
Butler & Tanner Ltd, Frome and London

Contents

Acknowledgments

I would particularly like to thank Lolly Stirk for her professional advice on the text and techniques, and for modelling for the drawings. I would also like to thank Eileen Fairbane for her early criticisms; Michael Burt and John Cooper for their instruction on body mechanics; Mary Stewart, Sandra Sabatini and Mina Semyon for their tireless and inspired yoga teaching; Beryl Sanders for the drawings; Caroline Taggart at Elm Tree Books for all her help and support; and Sports Locker: Notting Hill and Habit Mauritius for their tracksuits and T-shirts.

Introduction

FROM BIRTH, through infancy, the rough and tumble of childhood, youth, maturity and old age, the human structure is subject to falls, jars, blows, knocks, twists, stresses, strains, fatigue, postural conditioning, psycho-emotional traumas and extreme stimuli of one kind or another. As a result of this general wear and tear of life almost everybody displays a variety of asymmetries, imbalances and structural kinks. Individual symptoms may vary; low vitality, back pain, recurring strains, vague aches and pains with no apparent cause are just some of the signs that a body is tight, off balance and mechanically stressed. The prevention and treatment of this imbalance is called structural fitness.

What is structural fitness? What is meant by good body mechanics? Most of us are structurally and "bio-mechanically" unaware and tend to overlook the importance of the *framework* of the body for its own sake and in relation to all other aspects of health and well-being. We are used to thinking of the fit individual as someone who is slim, has neuro-muscular strength, circulo-respiratory endurance, stamina and a strong skeleton. Yet in spite of the "fitness revolution" of the last decade, structural disorders are as prevalent as ever. This view of fitness does not consider the advantages of a body with all its joints free and balanced, its muscles working in harmony; an integrated unit operating with minimal strain under all conditions. Yet all activity involves movement and the interaction of joints, and it is the quality of this movement and interaction that determines structural health.

Most of us experience some structural pain in our lives – sore backs, tight shoulders, stiff knees – but we are often unaware that the pain may be a result of a structural imbalance that has evolved over the years. Many structural faults are easily exaggerated or compounded, so some exercise can be worse than none at all. Many people who have been athletic in youth are surprised to find they have advanced wear and tear of their joints during middle or old age.

Our attitude to our own fitness may depend on our lifestyle. A dancer may be extremely fit but incapacitated by the occasional sprain or strain. On the other hand, an office worker's body may be rigid, off balance and lacking in fluidity, but he may have no aches and pains to speak of and feel his framework serves him well. Yet his poor structural condition may show up in patterns of fatigue, sensations of pressure, heaviness, tightness, unease and poor health generally. Many people don't realise that structure influences all the systems of the body – and its overall health.

Nowadays, more and more people are realising that the individual has a responsibility to care for his or her own health. It is becoming accepted that "therapies" should play a secondary role in health, and that education and prevention should play the primary role. However, there are still few organised systems that are directly concerned with the individual's need to change his or her own structure.

This book has grown out of a need: to clarify what constitutes sound structural exercise, what techniques meet everybody's mechanical needs, no matter what their individual ability. It has grown out of a demand. It teaches its reader how to change his or her body in a unique way. How to release and re-adjust it, simply and directly, free it up and balance it and in so doing improve overall health and well-being, remove physical and emotional stress, slow down the ageing process, and find less need to consult the help of structural therapists. Having studied, practised and taught both osteopathy and yoga for a number of years and having been confronted by people with all kinds of structural problems, experience tells me that there is a definite gap in our approach to health and fitness.

Furthermore, research shows that the structurally fitter individual can withstand fatigue for longer periods, is better equipped to tolerate physical stress, is more mentally alert, has a lesser degree of nervous tension, is emotionally more balanced, is less prone to injury, is less susceptible to infection and sickness, and is physically more confident. We *are* our structure, and structure is the essential physical feature of all human life.

You Are a Structure

THE HUMAN body is a structure made up of connected and dependent parts. Its basic framework consists of bone, cartilage, ligament, tendon and muscle. It is flexible, dynamic and subject to mechanical laws. The vital feature of the human structure is its joints and their integrity determines structural fitness. Where joints are stiff we must loosen them, where movement is lacking we must encourage it, where parts are compressed we must lengthen them, where they are too long we must shorten them. Only then, when the human structure is "freed up" and balanced at all its articulations can it be considered structurally and mechanically fit.

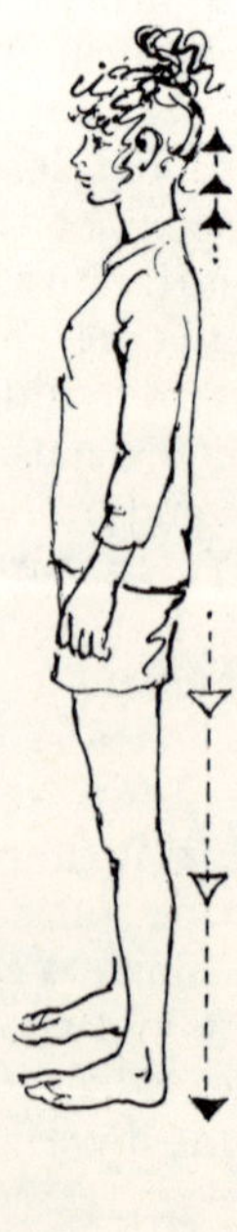

When the body is "freed up" and balanced it can be considered structurally and mechanically fit.

Your Structure is a Mechanism

THE JOINTS of the body continually interact, are all dependent on each other in some way and operate as a total mechanism. For example, the simple action of turning your head includes subtle movements of the entire spine. Even breathing involves a wave-like motion up and down the spinal column that includes all its joints. The joints of the feet interact with those connecting the neck and head during standing and walking. We are usually unaware of this subtle interaction, this fine adjustment between the different parts of the body, but it is going on all the time.

The body cannot adjust easily and economically when any of its joints are stiff, fixed or off balance. For example, stiffness in the hips causes a maladjustment between the pelvis and the spine, which puts strain on the spine. Restrictions in the feet can cause maladjustment and strain in the pelvis. Stiffness in the shoulders puts strain on the upper back and ribs, and so on. There are endless varieties of similar patterns that can exist in any one body.

However, we can "re-adjust" the body in order to improve its mechanics, its structure, and its capacity to self-adjust. Structural fitness demands three qualities. Firstly, each joint "space" should be under minimal compression during normal conditions i.e. the body must have the capacity to lengthen fully. Secondly, each joint should have its full natural range of movement. And thirdly the natural muscle pulls around each joint should be more or less balanced to keep its weight centred. If we stripped the skeleton of all its muscles, ligaments, and soft tissues and just left the bones they would fit together perfectly. The body is naturally and mechanically designed to self-adjust with the minimum of strain, friction and resistance between its parts. It is muscles that distort, inhibit and "bind" it up.

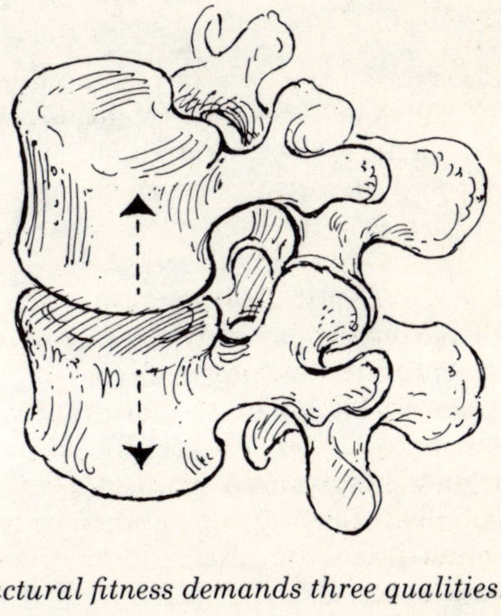

Structural fitness demands three qualities.

The Structural Epidemic

WHAT GRADUALLY stiffens and tightens the body? What upsets its natural balance? Why are so many of us, exercisers and non-exercisers, structurally unfit to a greater or lesser degree? There are various causes. The main offenders are gravity, poor posture, injury, disease, over-exercise, wrong exercise, no exercise, emotional disturbance, toxins, ageing, plus the extraordinary fact that the majority of structural faults go unnoticed and lie dormant for long periods with no apparently related ill effects. It is only when structure "breaks down" and pain or unease impair normal functioning that faults come to our attention.

Gravity

Gravity is the most potent physical influence in any human life; it is relentless, continually compressing, stretching, twisting, bending and distorting our bodies to some extent. Yet gravity is a phenomenon we rarely think about, it is there, we are earthbound and accept it. During normal activity we are not consciously aware of our own weight. When we are physically tired, sluggish or inert, we don't say that gravity has got the better of us; the feeling registers as fatigue, sluggishness or inertia and we express it so. However, our ability to carry our own weight with the minimum of strain is a basic feature of structural fitness. If your body weight is 65 kilogrammes, you don't feel it, that is you don't feel as if you are carrying 65 kilogrammes around with you. But if you pick up someone else of the same weight, it demands great effort to support the weight for any length of time. This same weight is acting on your body, is transmitted through your structure and falls through your joints for most of your active life. Gravity is solely responsible for postural strain and we must learn to respond effectively and adjust to its force. Gravity can drag us down into physical unease, ill health and strain, but it can also encourage our body to lengthen and release and reinforce our activities. When structure is free and balanced it responds to the force of gravity by lengthening, a sort of rebound effect. The downward pull of gravity is effectively met by the upward thrust from the ground. When this happens gravity nourishes structure instead of punishing it.

Posture is Dynamic

Posture is not an ideal word, but we haven't found a better one to date. It implies a position in space that is static. Posture is never completely static; the human framework is dynamic, constantly adapting and adjusting itself to the forces imposed upon it from moment to moment. Even when you are standing still, sitting still or lying down various parts of your framework are moving in relation to one another. The process of breathing itself involves bones moving in space. These movements may be rhythmically balanced and in harmony or may be fragmented, interrupted and disharmonious depending upon the fitness of the structure. Most of us have dynamic postural defects, rhythms out of sync due to stiffness, inflexibility and lack of resilience in our joints. Structural disharmony can exist on any level and the subtle imbalances are the most difficult to detect. Nevertheless they all influence structural health.

Lack of normal movement anywhere in the body can affect dynamic posture due to the total interdependence of all its moving parts. All the joints of the body need to participate in any movement and should not be held rigidly in a pattern unrelated to the task of the moment. The majority of postural imbalances great or small are due to rigidity somewhere in the structure. There are a whole variety of possible imbalances: feet too flat or too arched, legs rotated too far in or too far out, knock-knees, tilts and shunts of the pelvis, sideways curvatures and twists of the spine, exaggerated spinal curves and curves that are too straight or a combination of both. There are pigeon chests, protruding ribs, round shoulders, high shoulders, heads poking forward, heads pulling back and so on. Most of us have major or minor variations of these defects, though we may not notice subtle problems and may accept the more apparent ones as a fact of life and make no effort to correct them. Yet almost all the above conditions can be treated or prevented to some degree. When a body is obviously crooked it may not always be possible to change its appearance dramatically, but its fluidity and quality of movement can be improved.

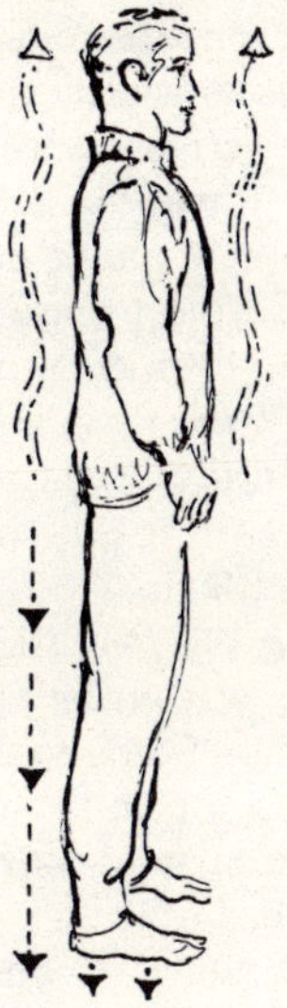

Posture is dynamic.

Structure and Injury

Many injuries have long term effects on structure. The scar tissue and muscular contraction that remain long after trauma and injury has resolved themselves can easily upset the mechanical balance of the body. Most of us have experienced the fact that muscles tighten and tense immediately in response to trauma. The area is naturally "splinted" against movement which may cause further damage. But it is the after-effect of many injuries that throws the mechanical balance of the body. For example an old ankle injury may leave it stiff and off balance. You may notice that when sitting on your heels on the floor you are lopsided because of the ankle's reluctance to extend fully, or discomfort may occur in the joint after a long walk, a run or a game of tennis. Such an ankle can cause strain and imbalance higher up in the body which may eventually surface as a knee, hip, lower back, shoulder or neck problem. It may even be responsible for severe headaches.

The residue of all trauma, great and small, can influence structural balance and rhythm. For example, nature responds to a bone fracture by laying down new cells around the entire fracture site. In turn the proliferating cells lay down a substance which calcifies and then organises into woven bone. Calcification has a thickening and hardening effect on the soft tissue around the site and this has mechanical repercussions such as local stiffness or muscle imbalance if the site is near a freely movable joint.

Soft tissue injuries to muscle, tendon, ligament and cartilage in the form of sprains, strains, tears, dislocations, lockings etc, all have long-term influence on body mechanics. Muscles surrounding a joint contract when any of its tissues are injured. When the initial injury resolves and the spasm subsides a residual contraction is left behind. When muscles remain excessively contracted for some time their structure changes and they become hard, stringy and lose their resilience. This process is called replacement fibrosis. It alters large and small muscles around joints and ultimately mechanical freedom and structural balance. The swelling and inflammation that often accompanies injury also leaves its mark. When swelling subsides the joints remain congested and gummed up for some time. This can lead to adhesions (adhere—to stick) and unless provisions are made to "mobilise" the joints, these adhesions eventually become fibrous and restrict free movement.

Some injuries are so minor and the initial recovery so quick that they simply register as the odd ache or pain in passing. This is especially common in the spine. The effects of some jars and shocks may go completely unnoticed, but all eventually exact a penalty on mechanical freedom. Adhesions, fibrosis and stiffness can affect the joints of the athlete, the keep-fitter and the non-exerciser alike. Whatever the circumstances the common denominator is the fact that structural trauma disorganises mechanical balance and freedom locally and throughout

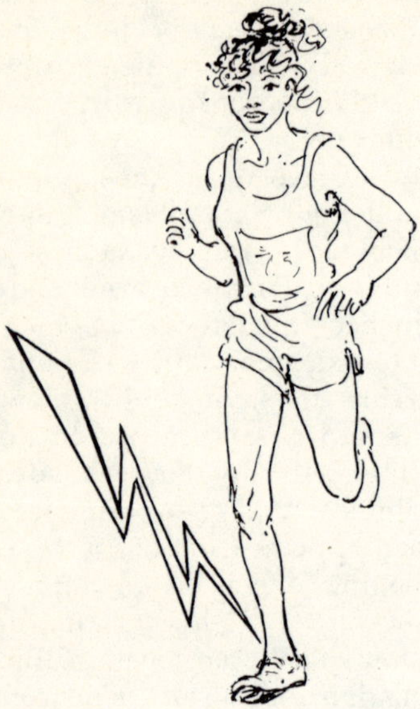

Old injuries upset structural balance.

the body as a whole. Even though some injuries are unavoidable and part of life, you can help prevent many of them by improving structural fitness and resilience. You can also work towards dissolving the long-term effects of injuries already sustained.

Structural Wear and Tear

The high incidence of wear-and-tear arthritis—now more commonly called Degenerative Arthrosis (DA)—is proof enough that we mismanage ourselves structurally. Various diseases and disorders affect structure, but DA is the most common and the one most related to mechanical stress. Wear and tear of joints is probably the oldest disorder known to man. Arthritic changes have been found in fossilised bones of dinosaurs: the ape man of the Pliocene Age and neolithic man of a later period suffered from joint degeneration; and Socrates listed arthritis as the most common disease of his time. Today millions suffer from DA and it is the most common condition met by orthopaedic physicians, osteopaths and chiropractors. Everyone who lives long enough gets some degree of DA. It is rare in people under 35, common over 65, and statistics show that *all* X-rays of the spines of people over 40, whether suffering from symptoms or not, show degenerative changes. The final changes occur in the cartilage, which dries out and eventually cracks, roughens and weakens. This basic material of the joints, their lining and shock-absorber, literally wears out, and this eventually affects the underlying bone. The quality of cartilage is influenced by various factors but the over-riding one seems to be strain arising from postural imbalances, poor body mechanics and wrong or excessive use. DA may exist in a joint but only become painfully apparent after a sudden injury. Many people with DA are unaware they have it and it is common for a routine X-ray to show extensive joint changes in people suffering no pain. The paradox is that because cartilage has relatively few pain-sensitive nerve-endings, it can wear away without causing discomfort until the condition has become quite advanced. DA presents most of a problem in weight-bearing joints and joints most frequently used. The overweight person may have it in the knees, labourers in the lower back, desk workers in the neck and upper back, and runners and hurdlers may develop changes in the hips later in life. People in this last category are often surprised to find they have developed DA as they spent much of their younger life doing athletics. Stiffness is the most common symptom, particularly after rest. The joints and surrounding tissues often 'set' like jelly and the muscles stiffen as a form of protection. Degeneration leads to stiffness, and in turn stiffness leads to more degeneration, a vicious circle. Wear-and-tear arthritis is the one joint disorder most likely to be prevented, or at least its onset delayed, by the individual working towards an acceptably fit structure. A finer mechanical balance in the body provides it with the ability to cope satisfactorily with all the stresses that hasten joint degeneration.

Structure, Stress and Exercise

The fitness revolution of the last decade, emphasising "get fit, keep fit, and stay fit", has been accompanied by some controversy. Certain forms of exercise recommended by cardiac specialists have been criticised by structural specialists, on the grounds that some of the activities used to push up cardiovascular fitness did so at the expense of structural fitness. For example, the aerobics bubble burst when people began to sustain a variety of injuries attributed to strain during class work. This led to the introduction of "low impact" aerobics. There is no doubt that exercise per se in the correct dosage is good for you in one way or another. But there is also no doubt that some exercise, if overdone or performed with a structure that is mechanically out of tune, hastens wear and tear. Many people subject their muscles and joints to extraordinary stress in the name of getting fit, losing weight, hardening muscle, firming up and getting a sweat going.

Two basic stresses act on the body at all times and are exaggerated during exercise. They are compressional stress—pressure or pushing together; and tensile stress—stretching or pulling apart. The elastic quality of our structure usually allows the exaggeration of compression and stretching for a short time and then a return to normal. Even under great stress for short periods our tissues lose shape and then return to normal when the stress is removed. But when the body is mechanically off balance, when normal stresses are already poorly tolerated, the added stress imposed by exercise leads to structural stiffness, strain and often injury. All activities exaggerate both compression and tensile stress, some more than others. Generally speaking, activities like running, jogging, tennis, squash and some class work exaggerate compression stress. Successive impact on the ground or floor and the jarring force of "putting on the brakes" can eventually lead to a reduction in the range of movement and compound any existing faults and imbalances in the feet, ankles, knees, hips and spine. You may be able to run ten miles and still be structurally unfit. Plenty of people jog, circuit train, play tennis or squash with stiff backs, round shoulders, tight ankles and so on. Martial arts, dancing and some aerobic classes exaggerate both stresses but tensile stress in particular. The martial artist with tight hips may overstretch his lower back or pelvic joints during a high kick. Forceful forward bending and side bending of the trunk during aerobics may have similar consequences. Because regular exercisers use their limbs far more than sedentary people, they increase the misuse of their tissues which can result in intermittent exaggerated stresses called micro-trauma. Many professional athletes and dancers remain in their prime for only a short time and their careers are often cut short because they overwork their structure.

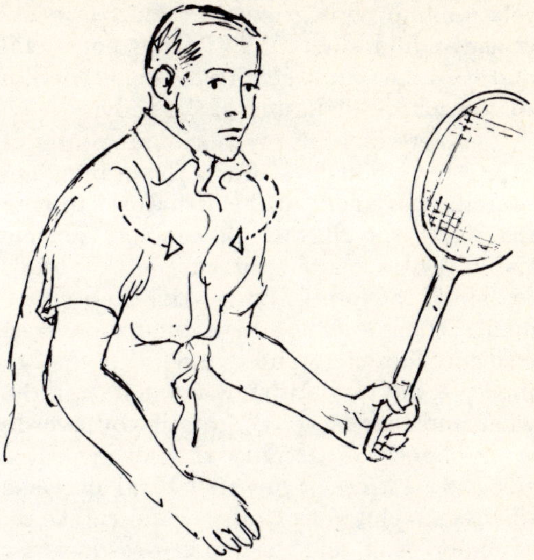

A tennis player with round shoulders will always have round shoulders.

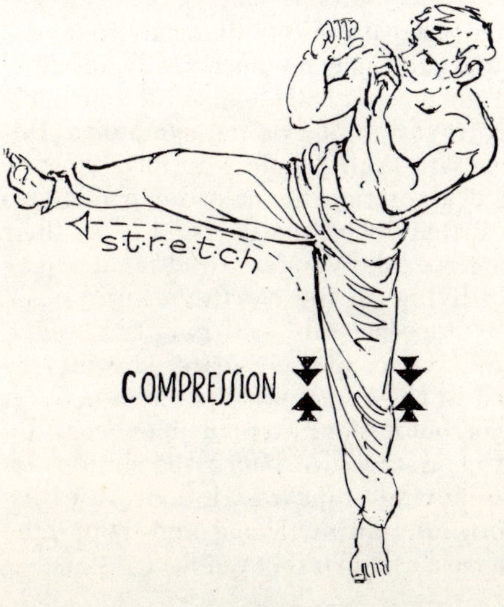

Two stresses are exaggerated during exercise.

However, most exercise does not claim to change structure or de-stress it in the mechanical sense. Most exercise does little to change the relationship between the parts of the body, its structural balance. A tennis player with round shoulders will always have round shoulders. A golfer with a short neck, elevated shoulders and a hunched upper back will always have a short neck, elevated shoulders and a hunched upper back. The runner with tight hips, knees and ankles will always have tight hips, knees and ankles. Exercise that is designed to change structure radically is confined to that alone. But if we can maintain a healthy relationship with gravity, if we are mechanically fluid, then all activity is beneficial and even the simple act of walking is enough to nourish the structure of the body.

Complete lack of any reasonable form of exercise obviously stiffens the joints and inhibits movement of the structure. During inactivity the fibrous elements of muscle tissue contract and shorten and this tends to "bind" the joints and restrict their movement. From the structural point of view exercise may loosen you up to a point if you are inactive, but may stiffen you and hasten the wear and tear of your joints if you overdo it or choose an activity that exaggerates structural stress. True structural exercise involves techniques that use the right mix of compression and stretch stresses in order to free and balance the body.

Structure and Food

Both the quality and the quantity of what we put inside ourselves influence structure. Our system throws out any excess of harmful toxins and waste products to the joints of the body in order to safeguard the vital organs. Toxic residue from metabolising certain foods actually clogs the joints and tissues and inhibits mechanical freedom; it is a factor in stiffness, the onset of arthritis and premature structural ageing. People who are structurally sensitive report a stiffening after-effect from eating or taking certain substances. The main offenders are things generally recognised as harmful: coffee, tea, alcohol, meat, sugar and tobacco.

Stopping the intake of certain things increases a sense of mechanical ease. Those who fast periodically claim that at a given point during the fast the system clears. A noticeable side-effect is the reduction of ongoing structural aches and pains. People who work on structure, who are structurally in tune, report that abstinence from food often results in a breakthrough with their structural "blocks". But one cannot fast indefinitely in order to maintain a higher degree of physical ease, and for most people it is almost impossible to stick to a limited and healthy intake for a sustained period without digressing. However if you are trying to improve mechanical fitness, you will achieve better results by maintaining a clean structure. This may involve a clean and varied diet, moderation in drinking and smoking and now and again leaving out all together those substances that release a high toxic residue into the body.

It is widely accepted that the *quantity* of food we eat influences body mechanics. Overweight generally causes strain on the weight-bearing joints and stiffens them, and a local distension of the digestive organs caused by over-eating can lead to strain on the lower back and pelvic joints.

Some people exercise in order to compensate for over-indulgence and this simply wears out the structure more rapidly and depletes vital energy. Moderation most certainly helps structure, but it is also true that moderate indulgences can be rendered relatively harmless by working on structure, as structural improvement tends to keep joints and muscles cleaner by its effect on digestion, metabolism and circulation.

Structure and Climate

There is no conclusive scientific evidence that climatic conditions effect the function of normal joints. However, the effect of climate on rheumatic and arthritic symptoms is legendary. Cold damp conditions exaggerate joint disorders and warm dry weather relieves them. A survey in Jamaica revealed a prevalence of rheumatic diseases similar to that of Britain, but people complained less. We all feel stiffer in the cold and damp and often old aches and pains may surface as a result. This is probably due to a narrowing of the blood vessels supplying the muscles and joints, and it is also believed that the viscosity of joint fluid may be raised. Cold and damp may not necessarily have any long-term mechanical effects over and above the aggravation of existing symptoms. But having said that, people who have spent a great deal of time in cold damp climates often display a particular rigidity in their movements. Many elderly and middle-aged people living on the North Atlantic coast exhibit an especially stiff gait that seems well in advance of their years. This may be related to the climate of their region, or it may not, but it is quite a plausible theory. By working on structure, improving circulation and removing joint restrictions, the discomforts of continual cold and damp conditions are considerably reduced.

Structure and Ageing

The changes of old age are to some extent inevitable but we can delay them. Ageing involves changes in the blood vessels, glands, and all the organs and tissues of the body. The systems of the body and their functions gradually run down. These changes are greatly influenced by changes in structure and by using structure as our main tool we can turn things around and delay the ageing process with remarkable results.

As a rule the ageing process is most apparent in its effect on the framework of the body. Postures and movements of the elderly are usually unmistakably stiff and rigid. Ageing decreases the distensibility of connective tissue and stiffens joints to the extent that sudden twists, jerks and movements can easily produce pain and cause irritation. Lubricating cells and tissues dry up, harden, contract, become more rigid and less elastic. Compressional strain is reflected in the narrowing of the joint spaces and people usually age in a flexed attitude i.e. knees bent, hips bent, the spine generally in a fixed position of forward bending and the shoulders curving forward on the rib cage. The joints become "set" in this familiar posture and the cartilage of the hips, knees and ankles softens because of wear and tear and abnormal joint mechanics. The spinal discs harden; changes in their surrounding ligaments can inhibit nerve impulses from the spinal cord to vital organs and tissues throughout the body and influence their competence.

However, there are many remarkable old people around. This may be due to their spirit, or to provisions made when younger through exercise, diet and lifestyle, or to regular activities kept up throughout old age. Nevertheless, people who age *really* well have aged well structurally and have usually spent many years involved in activities that encourage freedom and balance in the body. There are yoga teachers in their 70s with a fluidity of movement, posture, a bright-eyed and vital look, youthfulness, buoyancy and lightness that could be envied by someone 25 years their junior. Maintaining a healthy structure is a fundamental measure towards delaying all the disorders common to old age. Not only is it possible to prevent arthritis and wearing of the joints, but a free and balanced structure provides an environment for all the machinery of the body to thrive well into old age. Good posture and freedom of movement aids blood and nerve supply to and from all vital organs and tissues, keeps them free from unnecessary pressure and gives them adequate support. Free interplay within joints and mechanical balance is an index to health and an investment for the later years.

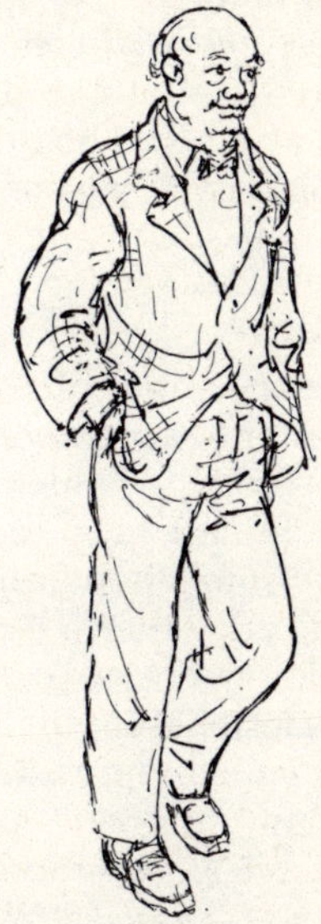

People who age really well have aged well structurally.

Structure and Emotions

Our emotional life has an enormous impact on our structure. Every thought and feeling registers in our muscles and joints and our emotional structure and our physical structure blend to form who we are, and how we act and react. We all have a physical personality that matches our personality in general, all our behaviour is expressed through our structure and personalities can be analysed by their structural behaviour. When we find it inappropriate to express certain feelings we suppress them by muscular contractions. These contractions are responsible for holding in feelings: we call this tension.

There are two degrees or types of muscle tension related to our emotional life. Temporary tension involves tensing up in response to immediate situations and includes moment-to-moment changes in muscle tone, holding the breath, tightening the belly, lifting the shoulders and so on.

Sometimes we are aware of these responses in ourselves and sometimes they remain beneath the conscious level. There are also deep, "bound in" chronic tensions and contractions that develop from an early age as part of the personality. They result from the chronic suppression of feelings and are normally unconscious; they become second nature and part of our character. Both forms of muscular tension relate to each other and both affect posture, attitudes, movements, mechanical freedom and balance of the structure as a whole and health in general. But the chronic type of tension is by far the more insidious and physically disruptive.

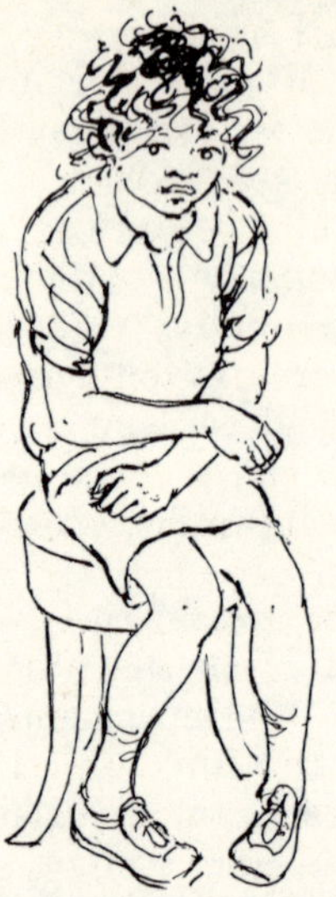

Reich was interested in the WAY feelings were suppressed.

Chronic Tension

There is a process familiar to psychoanalysts that to a greater or lesser extent occurs in all of us. A process which enables us to behave "normally" by holding in feelings, a process by which we stop ourselves falling apart and hold ourselves together. Psychoanalysis shows that the majority of its patients experiencing emotional conflicts have undergone a process called repression. That is, at certain points in childhood, patients have suppressed, held back, held in and cut off to various emotional impulses. Wilhelm Reich over forty years ago was the first to make extensive studies of the fact that the skeletal muscles played a key role in the suppression of these impulses. He called this process "muscular armouring", implying that one armoured oneself against overwhelming sensations. In *The Function of the Orgasm* (Pocket Books) he wrote, "In the final analysis I could not rid myself of the impression that somatic (physical) rigidity represents the most essential part in the process of repression. All our patients report that they went through periods in childhood, in which by means of certain practices (holding the breath, tensing the abdominal muscular pressure) they learned to suppress their impulses of hate, anxiety and love. Until now, analytic psychology has merely concerned itself with *what* the child suppresses and with *what* the motives are which cause him to control his emotions. It did not enquire into the *way* in which children habitually fight against impulses. It is precisely the physiological process of repression that deserves our keenest attention. It never ceases to be surprising how the loosening of a muscular spasm not only releases the vegetative energy, but over and above this reproduces a memory of that situation in infancy in which the repression of the instance occurred. It can be said that every muscular rigidity contains the history and the meaning of its origin. It is not as if we had to derive from dreams or associations how the muscular armour developed. The armour is the form in which the infantile experience is preserved as an impairment of functioning." Reich related various physical attitudes, fixations and rigidities to the chronic and ultimately unconscious suppression of impulses over the years, to the extent that they become part of the person, part of the character. For example, the jaw and throat may stiffen as a result of continually holding back the impulse to cry. Muscles of the chest and neck may become chronically stiff in continued efforts to suppress feelings of anxiety. Muscles of the pelvis and thighs may eventually harden and shorten as a result of repeated efforts to suppress unwanted sexual feelings. Reich also observed that there was no neurotic individual who did not show a tension in the abdomen, and he noted the common tendency of people to hold their breath and inhibit exhalation as a means of controlling their feelings.

Since Reich, other authorities have taken this phenomenon even further. Those involved in the Body-Mind work essentially coming out of the west coast of America have taken to analysing personalities in great detail by the way they appear structurally and suggest that emotional splits and conflicts relate to physical patterns on a very specific level. It has been suggested for example that flat feet indicate one is emotionally ungrounded. Clutching feet with a high arch and gripping toes are equated with an unresolved conflict involving the impulse to run away. It has been suggested that ankle and knee stiffness is related to conflicts around feelings of pride and progress. A pelvis tipped up at the front supposedly implies a holding in of sexual feelings and the opposite implies a heightened energy and flow. Chronic tightness in the buttocks is related to an attitude of forcefully holding on to all expressions, feelings and creative instincts. Tension in the pelvic floor relates to controlling one's position in life and also restricts sexual feeling. The abdominal cavity is supposed to be the most vulnerable and unprotected body-mind region, as this is where many emotions and passions originate and a lifetime of firmly holding on to one's feelings gets locked up here. Feelings of anger, rage, unhappiness, violence, tearfulness, loneliness and sorrow may be held in the belly. It is suggested that the lower back area acts as a psychosomatic mediator between the top and bottom halves of the body. Feelings and pressures such as demands of authority, duty and guilt, coming from above, meet feelings of self-support, self-control, sexuality and stability, coming from below. The lower back is a primary site for conflict between these feelings.

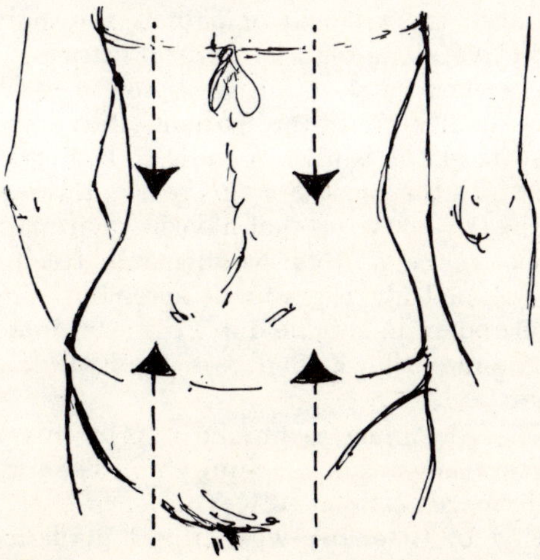

The lower back acts as a psychosomatic mediator between the top and bottom halves of the body.

Chest contraction may indicate a passive personality with feelings of depression and a chronic sense of inferiority. The large overgrown expansive chest indicates a blown-up ego. Round shoulders carry the weight of the world on them, raised shoulders indicate fear, forward shoulders a fear of being hurt and pulled back shoulders the attempt to keep one's temper and resist the impulse to strike out at the world. The upper back holds anger and the head too far forward on the neck indicates great caution. A tight throat relates to fear of expression. The bottom of the jaw holds anger and impulses to bite and cry, a receding jaw reflects the suppression of screaming, a protruding jaw, defiance and aggression. A clenched jaw suggests great self-control and the holding in of all expression, and facial tension results from conflicts to do with who we pretend to be and how we pretend to be feeling towards others.

Our emotional history is undoubtedly anchored in our structure. We remain chronically angry or whatever because the emotion is still fixed in the body. We all have deep-rooted tensions and we can certainly relate them to emotional patterns if we want to. By necessity we do learn to hold our tensions in, perhaps anywhere or everywhere in the body. It might be healthier in some respects to cry, scream and release our innermost feelings spontaneously in response to the stress of life and this might result in our being emotionally and structurally more balanced. But unless we all become more tolerant of each other, such behaviour is unlikely to be well received by those around us. If we want to "dig deeply" we should seek the appropriate help from analysts who are professionally experienced in this work. There are, however, many people with flat feet, tipped pelvises, round shoulders, etc, who lead to all intents and purposes satisfactory lives and are successful in their own terms.

Nevertheless, improving one's own physical structure does help emotional balance. Daily tensions that arise are removed quite easily, and deeper tensions release slowly as structure improves. The advantage here is that old emotions and wounds are not suddenly released into consciousness, flooding one with overwhelming sensations possibly bottled up since childhood. By working on your own structure you release the deeper tensions and move towards an emotional balance at a pace that is level with the pace of the structural balance and freedom achieved. Very often the person improving his or her structure is unaware of old emotional wounds and scars easing. Such changes may simply register as the odd dream related to childhood and the occasional insight. At its simplest, emotional balance related to structural improvement is explained as a greater sense of emotional ease, spontaneity and relaxation. Even with successful techniques we don't free ourselves from all our muscular tensions, since the condition of life itself constantly imposes a state of tension upon us. Those with the ideal structure are not free from emotional stress, but the minimum of tension needed to respond to any given situation must be preferable to the chronic tensions resulting from a lifetime of inhibited expression. As structure balances, emotional turmoil can and does settle.

Structure, Responsibility and Education

The widespread prevalence of structural kinks, stiffness, rigidities, asymmetries and imbalances is mainly due to the fact that most people regard faulty structures as normal. We only take an interest in structure when it breaks down; consequently factors such as gravity, poor posture, emotional tensions, ageing and so on go unchecked, they get a grip and they take hold. This is a social phenomenon: society is basically *bio-mechanically* unaware. We *allow* structural strain and disorganisation to set in to the extent that it does.

We are usually unaware of our structural faults and kinks until something goes wrong, such as the painful experience of "putting something out" or "pulling something", often during normal activity. This rebellion of the body is usually the final stage of a long process of underlying imbalance. Even with all the current emphasis on health and fitness, structure is rarely tested. If someone can do all he has to do in relative comfort, why bother to go and have all his joints tested? If that someone uses about a hundred words in his language we say he is mentally deficient. Yet the majority of us use only a few variations of about a hundred or more of the body's two thousand possible movements and most of these tend to be restricted. But we would never take anyone seriously if they suggested that we were physically deficient. We may periodically have our heart and blood pressure checked as a matter of course, but rarely if ever our level of structural fitness. Medical assessments don't usually include a structural assessment, probably because structural fitness is not considered essential to life. Obviously the healthy function of the heart and other organs is a major concern, but the fact that structural function also indirectly affects all the systems of the body is largely overlooked. We are resigned to a general level of structural health that is well below par and when structure rebels we put ourselves in the hands of others. We give the responsibility to osteopaths, chiropractors, doctors, and various therapists, who spend the bulk of their time and energy treating the painful symptoms of poor body mechanics. They can sometimes remove pain and disability with remarkable results, and indeed we would be lost without their skill. However, true structural health does not depend on the use of treatment that comes from the outside, it depends on the proper management, use and movement of the body by the individual. Manipulative therapists excel at removing symptoms but have neither the time nor the technique to teach people how they can improve structure. Because the removal of pain is the main objective, long-term structural fitness is overlooked and often symptoms recur periodically, giving the "patient" the feeling that he or she is always going to be dependent on a therapist. For this reason interest in the few activities that have as their main objective a more total balance and "freeing up" of the body, is gradually spreading. The forerunners in this field are the Alexander technique, the Feldenkrais method, and yoga.

The Alexander technique is primarily a postural education, teaching you to use your body more economically. You learn over a period of time and with initial guidance from a teacher how to release unnecessary tension and to use your body with maximum mechanical efficiency, by conscious commands and directives that you give yourself constantly in order to balance posture and movements. Eventually this process becomes automatic and you just need the occasional "topping up" from a teacher.

The Feldenkrais method teaches body awareness through movement: its approach educates the nervous system to adopt more ease and economy of movement and in so doing removes structural strain.

Yoga is more widely known and although its physical techniques are but one facet of its philosophy and practice, it is unsurpassed in its approach to body mechanics—that is if you have a good teacher. If the exponents of these activities had their way the structural concept would become part of our culture and accepted as part of daily life.

All authorities on structural balance agree that our standard of and approach to physical education is largely to blame for the prevalence of structural disorders, and all believe that this education should begin in the early years of life. Many structural disorders encountered in adolescence and adulthood stem from strains and traumas that occur in early life. Many children display signs of stiff spines, tight hips, tense shoulders and a variety of postural defects. Even though most schools encourage games, sports and PE, they fail to meet the needs of many children in terms of their body mechanics. Neither Alexander, Feldenkrais, yoga or any other suitable system is available to children at school. This inevitably leads to the unchecked development of structural problems, the majority of which manifest themselves and surface later in life.

All children would benefit from a compulsory standardised system of structural exercise that was not competitive, and considered what was needed generally, with individual variations. It should be taught in groups accompanied by simple lessons in the *theory* of good body mechanics. Once this has been put into practice, games, sports and PE can be added. The solution is not to get rid of the sports and games, but to begin at the real starting point, begin with the body and then go on to the sport. This would lead to a great reduction in the prevalence of structural problems and bring the true feel of what it means to be structurally healthy within everyone's reach.

Structure and Inner Fitness

WE HAVE said that improving structure improves posture, slows down ageing and makes it more enjoyable, prevents arthritis, improves all exercise and movement and encourages emotional balance. People who spend time on structure also find they have obvious benefits such as fewer muscular aches and pains, greater physical ease and self-confidence; sleep improves and a greater sense of relaxation is achieved. But there are also other benefits related to the "inner fitness" of the body that often come as a surprise: benefits involving the inner organs, body awareness, energy levels and aerobic fitness.

Organic Fitness

Organic fitness basically means that the inner organs work better. Tendencies towards problems such as indigestion, constipation and menstrual pain seem to resolve themselves as structure changes. We function as a total organism and the function of one part cannot be separated from the function of another. The inner organs are dependent on each other and, working together, process fuel in the form of food and oxygen to drive and move the human machine. Structure depends on its inner organs but they too depend on structure. The framework of the body has a marked influence on the stomach, liver, spleen, pancreas, intestines, kidneys, bladder and the reproductive organs. Mabel Elsworth Todd, a pioneer of the structural concept, wrote in 1920, "Gravity is an elementary force, it acts upon structure as a whole and each separate part. Faulty adjustment in relationship to this causes interference with the proper reaction of articulated parts and free co-ordination of muscles. The deeper we study the subject of mechanics and posture, the more we realise how far-reaching this effect is upon the entire organism."

The early osteopaths maintained that because the body has no spare or unoccupied inner space, there is no physical room for any disturbance in the relationship of the inner organs. Organs that are misplaced through bad posture put tension and pressure on other organs and in turn are subject to the same influence. When pressure and strain on an organ is continued for long enough, it may cause permanent damage and result in a chronic condition. Usually this kind of disturbance comes slowly and the function of the organs changes only after years of faulty posture or poor body mechanics. The usual variety of imbalances may be responsible. Exaggerated spinal curves, tilted pelvis, round shoulders and even flat feet can all in some way exert pressure on the inner organs of the body.

It seems common sense to expect better health with the structure of the body in balance and with maximum mechanical freedom so that all the inner organs are free from pressure, overcrowding and distention.

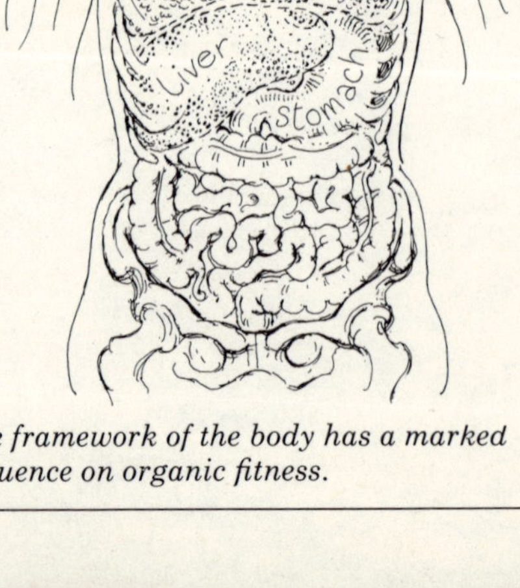

The framework of the body has a marked influence on organic fitness.

The beneficial effect of structural improvement on organic health is also borne out by the experience of many people who practise yoga. B. K. S. Iyengar, in his book *Light on Yoga*, gives groups of postures for various organic ailments. He bases his recommendations on 25 years' experience with his pupils. He suggests postures for various organic disturbances and includes routines for problems such as acidity, dyspepsia, heartburn, indigestion, colic, colitis, gastritis, constipation, flatulence, gastric ulcer, diabetes, displaced uterus, labour pains and menstrual and prostrate disorders, as well as general postures to influence the abdominal organs, spleen, pancreas, intestines, kidneys, gall bladder and liver.

Structure and Sensitivity

Body awareness, our kinaesthetic sense, is both conscious and unconscious. We can consciously feel and sense our physical selves, but at the same time the body's perception of information about muscle tension, movement, weight and position usually occurs beneath a conscious level. Our kinaesthetic sense is a background sense but even as such this sense may be gross, dull and blocked, or fine, keen and perceptive, depending upon the condition of the structure.

The nerve-endings responsible for this sense form a network throughout our muscles, tendons, joints and bones and inform the nervous system of changes and deviations occurring inside and outside the body. They respond to stretch and contraction and warn the muscles of dangerous levels of both. This sensory input and the responses to them are known as simple reflexes. Throughout the body, impulses of one kind (sensation and perception) are translated into impulses of another kind, action and movement. The central nervous system receives feedback concerning changes in muscle tension and ranges of movement so that it may adjust the body accordingly, the nature of the adjustment determined by the needs of the moment.

All our postures and movements are based on these reflexes. Even though to a large extent we are unaware of reflex activity, we often know if an action or a movement felt right, whether it felt smooth, easy and strain-free or unco-ordinated, tense and jerky. Either we have a good body awareness or we don't. But, because we act and react as a whole, we can influence the more unconscious side of our kinaesthetic sense by developing the more conscious side, by developing the "feeling" of our body. Tension, stiffness and rigidity greatly reduce the sensitivity of the structure. This is why so many people have tense muscles and stiffness in their joints and yet are unaware of it. Once an unnecessary contraction is established in a muscle its sensitivity, its ability to sense fine changes is impaired, it "feels" less. All sensing of muscular activity relies upon the smallest amount of residual contraction in the muscles and by reducing tension and tightness, by freeing structure, we can improve kinaesthetic sensation. There is no doubt that increasing mechanical freedom increases sensitivity: where there is more movement there is less tension. But it is the *approach* to movement that is so important in improving awareness. Repetitive movements lacking precision, concentration and attention have limited value in terms of sensitivity and may even block feeling in the body. There is a big difference between being aware of the body and have a good body awareness. We can be aware of our body in our head, as it were, and this is true of many people who exercise, who use their body athletically but are not really 'in touch' with it. However, by using the right approach we begin consciously to sense distorted patterns of posture and movement we may have been stuck with for years. To improve awareness and sensitivity we approach the body in a way that encourages the observation of "feeling". The movements are slow and enable us to shift the attention inwards; we discover ourselves from the inside. As we slowly adjust in a technique, the feeling of the relevant part of the body comes into consciousness.

Improving the kinaesthetic sense not only gives us more pleasure generally, but also enables us to sense strain in time to prevent injury and damage. Many injuries occur because we didn't sense the strain at the time. When the body is structurally free and balanced, the reflexes are sharper, the translation of sensation into action is more efficient and the spontaneous adjustments of the body from moment to moment are more harmonious.

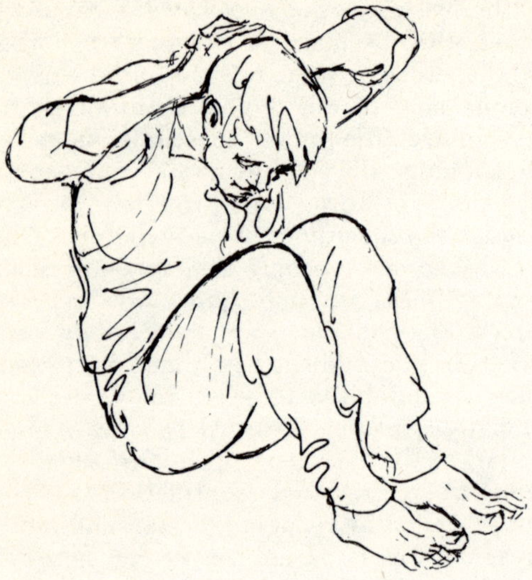

Repetitive movements may even block feeling in the body.

Structure and Energy

All our activity and our health in general are determined by our energy levels and rhythms. Energy can be classified as physical and mental but it is all the same energy. In whatever form our energy or lack of it is most apparent, its levels and rhythms are a considerable indication of our state of health and vitality. Life's energy courses through us, it circulates for better or worse in every living body and when it is blocked, depleted or fragmented, the organism suffers in one way or another.

All the systems of the body, glandular, nervous, digestive, circulatory, respiratory, reproductive, immune, and musculo-skeletal (structural), are involved in the production, maintenance, regulation and expenditure of energy. The condition of each system influences the vital energy of every other system and any one system functioning below par depletes the energetic state of the body and the person as a whole. Physiologists tell us that even in the fittest and most efficient human machine, only 15% of total energy is available for conscious purposes, 85% being used for the unconscious internal processes of the body. Any impairment in the unconscious processes requires new energy and can only draw on the 15% needed for the conscious activities of the day. In other words, energy depletion may occur beneath a conscious level but the effect is felt consciously and registers as low energy and fatigue.

Most of the energy produced and mobilised by the body is used to drive the structure, move the framework. Movement is the primary requirement for the continuation of life; without movement we are unlikely to survive and flourish. Structure is the main reason for energy expenditure and, conversely, structure has a remarkable influence on energy levels and rhythms.

Stiff joints and muscles block energy circulation; muscle tension is in fact energy bound up in muscle. Tension is a static muscular contraction that uses energy to grip bones and establish a sense of security both physically and emotionally. Static contractions seldom release completely and even in sleep the structure holds on. Excessive tension fragments the transfer of energy through the body, it ceases to flow freely, it gets dammed up and it deprives the entire organism of a free and healthy energetic flow.

Static tension also uses more energy in movement. Muscles must work to cause movement but their opposing muscles must also release sufficiently to allow ease of movement. Economy of effort demands movements that are made with the least resistance and minimal contraction. Where excessive tension exists, extra energy is used doing anything and everything from answering the phone to walking, to playing tennis, to simply sitting and giving something your attention, even to sleeping.

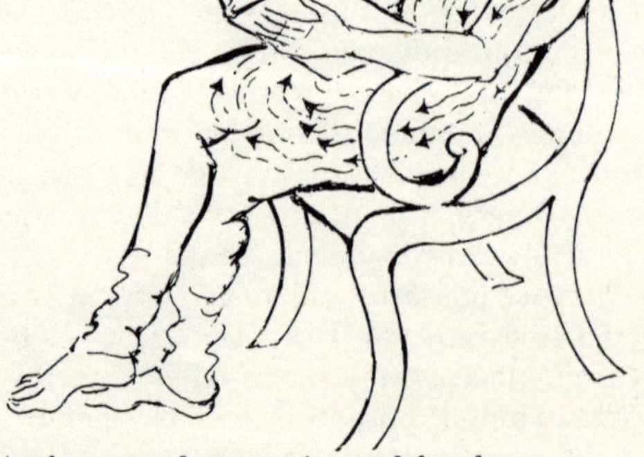

85% of our total energy is used for the unconscious internal processes of the body.

Blocked, wasted and depleted energy can lead to fatigue on any level and the organism as a whole may suffer. Some people believe that all illnesses are caused by disturbance in energy flow. The Taoist way of thinking calls the dynamic energy of the body "Chi" and its harmonious flow is thought to be the prime requirement for health. There is no doubt that once the structure becomes freer and more balanced it is much more economical in terms of its energy expenditure. When the body is more balanced and fluid, less energy is needed to move it and once blocks begin to dissolve more energy is released for use. As a result the entire organism benefits as energy is raised on all levels, conscious and unconscious.

Structure and Aerobic Fitness

All activity, life in fact, is aerobic because aerobic simply means living or taking place in the presence of air or oxygen. Aerobic fitness, however, is taken to mean the capacity for the heart, lungs and blood vessels (the circulo-respiratory system) to supply oxygen to and remove waste products from working muscles during strenuous exercise. Such exercise may include running, squash, tennis, cycling, swimming, aerobic classes, circuit training and so on. People who work regularly on their aerobic capacity are often surprised at the improvement they experience if they improve their structural fitness. They quickly realise how much their capacity improves due to the removal of the common structural blocks that impede breathing and circulation and waste valuable energy. The structurally fit individual improves aerobically on all levels because as structure changes the chest cavity relaxes and opens up more, the heart and lungs have maximum room in which to function, all the joints and muscles involved in breathing are mechanically free, there is less resistance to overall circulation, less resistance to movement and as body mechanics generally improve more vital energy is released for aerobic performances.

Breathing

There is more to the mechanics of breathing than most people imagine. Normal breathing involves not only movements of the rib cage but also movements of the entire spine. The spine lengthens from one end to the other during every inhalation and shortens during every exhalation. Air enters the lungs because the diaphragm opens the chest cavity and the intercostal (inter-rib) muscles open it from side to side and from back to front. This results in an air pressure less than that of the atmosphere so that outside air rushes in to equalise the pressure. Then the diaphragm and the intercostals relax, increasing the inside pressure and expelling the air. The joints and muscles of the shoulders, neck and pelvis also assist in this process.

In the more extreme activity of aerobic performances, all these structures work harder and faster and call on accessory muscles in the legs, arms and even the jaw to assist in the opening and closing of the chest cavity. Almost the entire human structure focuses on the sole and urgent purpose of expanding the chest in all directions. Even though the "effort" to breathe may persist, aerobic performance is much easier from the mechanical point of view when the spine, rib cage, shoulders and hips are free, in balance and interacting smoothly.

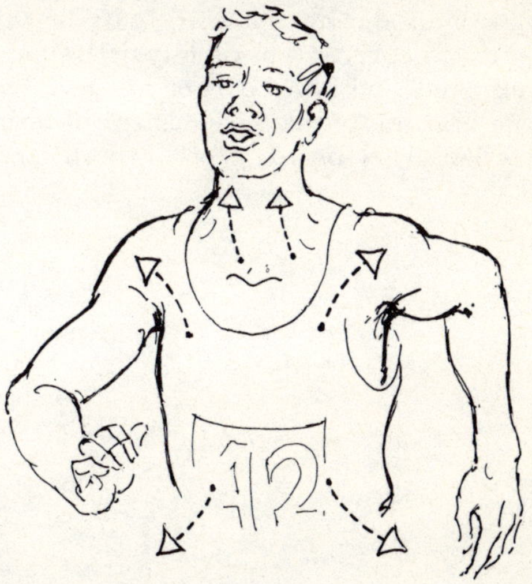

In aerobic performances almost the entire human structure focuses on the sole and urgent purpose of expanding the chest in all directions.

The Heart

The heart is a muscular pump expelling about five litres of blood per minute during rest and up to thirty-five litres per minute during exercise. As a working muscle it receives its own oxygen supply from blood transported from the lungs via the coronary arteries. Its demand for oxygen may increase four to five times during aerobic performances. From the mechanical point of view the position of the heart is important, it can vary slightly between individuals and it normally changes shape and position with each breath. Structural imbalances can therefore affect and put strain on the heart. Exaggerated and continual postural defects can compress the heart and may even displace it. Imbalances in the spine can put strain on the diaphragm on which the heart rests and so undermine its support. If the shoulders and ribs have a tendency to droop, the diaphragm is lowered and takes the heart with it. Exaggerated spinal curves also influence the heart's support and stiffness in the upper ribs may throw strain and pressure upon it. The effects of poor support, pressure or displacement are not immediately serious. No-one believes that stiff joints and poor posture would provoke a heart attack in the short term. But research shows that strain and pressure on the tissues surrounding and supporting the heart can influence its function in the long term. Osteopathic researchers during the early part of this century discovered that rigidity in the upper back joints and lower part of the neck had some bearing on the development of heart disorders. They proved experimentally that disturbances to the heart's direct nerve supply from these areas upset its rhythm and altered the quality of its muscle tissue.

Few people with a heart disorder would think of committing themselves exclusively to the care of an osteopath. But those changing their lifestyle under the care of a wholistic and naturopathic practitioner would probably find themselves being treated structurally during the course of their therapy. It would be impossible to prove that a healthy person who had his or her body "loosened" regularly by an osteopath in the name of good maintenance might have developed a heart disorder had he or she not followed such a course of action over the years. But having said this it is rare to find a yoga teacher of any age with a heart problem.

Circulation

Structure also influences the circulation of blood to and from working muscles. Since most blood vessels traverse, lie beneath or are surrounded by muscles, any over-contracted state of muscle is bound to squeeze the vessels and make it more difficult for the heart to pump blood through them. If muscles are tense, hard and fixed, their unchanging pressure makes it more difficult for blood to permeate the tissues, deposit

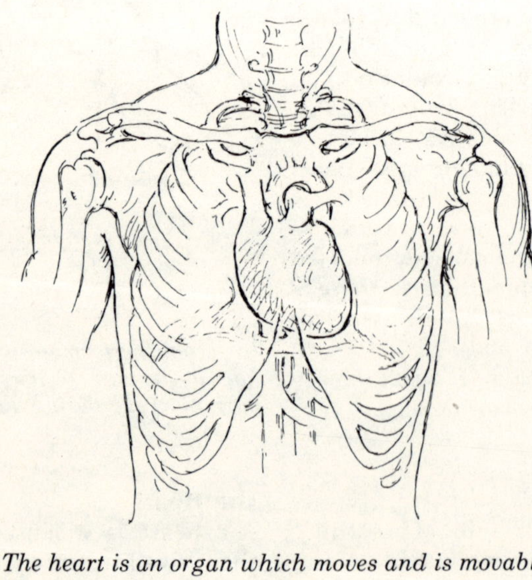

The heart is an organ which moves and is movable.

oxygen, pick up waste and return via the veins to the heart. This affects the chemical turnover in the muscle tissues and consequently impairs performance.

The most common experience shared by those who work on structure and do some kind of aerobic training is the marked feeling of increased energy and lightness while training. This is due to the fact that as structure frees and balances, the body works against less resistance to movement, and its ability to adjust spontaneously is more harmonious. All strain-free and efficient movement depends on good body mechanics. When activity is extreme, structural fitness is especially important, not only for the benefit of the joints and muscles but also so that the breathing and circulatory systems may work harmoniously and gain the greatest benefit from the exercise or activity.

Structure Piece by Piece

THIS SECTION highlights some pertinent facts concerning the freedom and balance of each part of the structure and its relation to the integrity of the body as a whole, and includes all the specific structural techniques.

The following advice on approaching the techniques should be read before trying them out. This is essential when practising any kind of body work from a book.

If you have a problem

All the techniques are perfectly safe in form and approach, but if you have a structural tendency that warrants particular caution it is advisable to consult your osteopath, chiropractor, physiotherapist or whoever understands your problem. Show them this book and tell them you plan to begin a structural fitness programme. If you have a structural imbalance that surfaces painfully on occasions, only practise during a pain-free period. If you have a lower back problem and are recovering from a recently painful episode, practise all the techniques in the back pain section (page 80) for at least a month before going through the main section and its routines.

Otherwise

Almost everyone gets the odd "twinge" here and there and now and again, so most people can start enjoying the techniques straight away. This book is for those who "think" they are structurally fit as well as those who know they are not.

The Approach

In prescribing techniques for this book, I have had to deal with the problem of either giving too much instruction and putting the reader off, or not giving enough so that the reader gets it wrong. In an effort to get it right and yet keep it simple, I have provided the minimum necessary instruction with the view that certain aspects of the techniques are clearly shown in the illustrations. *Study the illustrations carefully as well as reading the instructions.* Where the instruction falls a little thicker, it is worth remembering that you only have to go through a technique a few times to get the basics of it. After this only occasional reference to the instructions will be necessary and the illustrations should provide an adequate guide.

All the techniques decompress the joints, balance out muscle pulls, promote a fuller range of movement and generally release structure. They are a mix of stretch, release, stabilising and visualisation techniques. There are techniques for each part of the structure followed by routines that bring it all together and integrate the body as a whole.

Grades

Some techniques you will find easy and others may take longer to develop. Many are graded and once the body starts to "free" you can move on to the next grade. Some techniques have two or three grades, a few have four or five, and some are not graded and are immediately suitable for everyone. Where the techniques are graded always try grade one before going on to the next grade and only then when you can manage the previous one without strain. *This may take time,* but the quality and the fineness of movement is more important and more productive than forcing ranges of movement or straining too hard. Don't worry if you seem to be stuck around a grade one or two technique. Progression to grades three or four is not always essential or even possible for some people. You can maintain an above average degree of structural fitness by regularly practising the non-graded and the grade one and two techniques. If you could maintain this standard alone through middle and old age, it would still be remarkable by normally accepted standards. Those familiar with aerobics, yoga or dance may move straight into grades three or four, and some of the techniques may be familiar. But the subtleties of each technique may be new and the concept of imaging and visualising movement in various positions certainly provides a valuable and for some people unexplored means of improving structure whatever their standard or ability.

Gross and Subtle

At first sight the basic movements and positions—their gross aspect—are obvious. Techniques that simply appear to lengthen the spine or bend the hips, do just that. But, each technique also has its subtle aspect, and this is all-important if change is to be progressive and lasting. This aspect involves small, conscious adjustments in each technique, such as subtle broadenings, lengthenings, softenings or sensing heaviness, release or relaxation. The subtle concept should be taken seriously: gross movements are not enough on their own. We need subtlety to be able to direct and adjust the body from the inside. Suggest to the body that change is possible. Concentrate on *releasing* muscles, not forcing them. The subtleties of self-adjustment become more apparent as time goes by. Be inventive in each technique, get to know your own body and your own structural subtleties by yourself and for yourself. This book is just a door between yourself and all kinds of possibilities—open it.

Practical tips

- Always work bare foot.
- Regular practice if only for a short time is more beneficial than an occasional blitz. Four half-hour or two one-hour sessions a week should be adequate to start with.
- Don't work with a full stomach.
- Always wear loose comfortable clothing. Tight leotards can restrict movement and inhibit your ability to sense the finer aspects of good structural work.
- Follow the arrows in the illustrations. They show lines and directions of movement that you should be thinking and moving in. For example, in the following illustration arrows A and B suggest a feeling of width across the shoulders. Arrow C suggests consciously dropping the tail bone and arrow D suggests feeling a sense of weight through the heels.

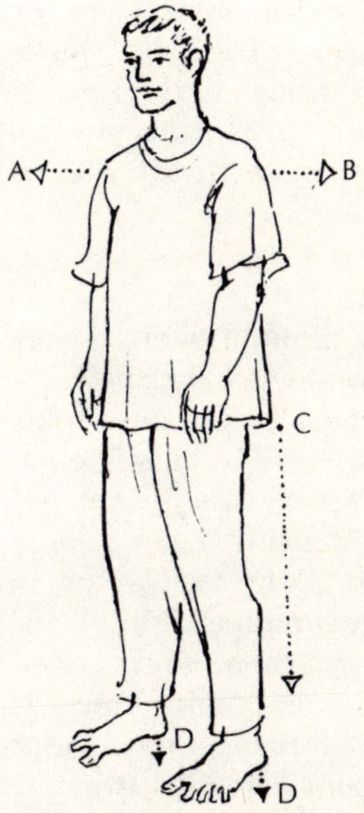

Assistance

Some techniques use the help of a chair, wall, table, book, strap, folded towel, blanket, cushion or another person. Working with a mirror can sometimes be useful to compare your own positioning, grading and general progress with the illustrations and to check your symmetry.

Sensation

The sensation produced by each technique will vary from person to person. *Don't put yourself through pain.* A good strong sensation of stretch and sometimes contraction is often needed and is productive, but it should not be so strong that you cannot relax, release, adjust and where necessary imagine movement at the same time. This is impossible if you tense up against a forced or painful movement. Be particularly cautious of undue pain in the knees and lower back.

However, one needs a certain amount of resistance to "bite on". It is usually the feeling of resistance and stiffness in particular techniques that highlights our specific imbalances and blocks. A moderate or strong sensation of stretch is acceptable if you can consciously release the resistance, soften the sensation and begin to dissolve the block. In many of the techniques you can concentrate on the sensation of stretch and contraction while developing a sense of the subtleties at the same time. For example, you can concentrate on the sensation of stretch at the back of the knees in a forward bend while cultivating an awareness of what's happening in the feet, pelvis, spine and shoulders.

Visualisation

The power of mind over body is legendary. Our minds can make our bodies sick and can also cure them. By the same token minds can tighten structure but also help to release it. If you can accept this you can help to change structure by using a few simple mind's-eye techniques along with the freeing and releasing techniques. It has been shown that you can lengthen your spine simply by imagining it is lengthening. Visualisation can to a degree change the relationship between bones and lengthen and release joints and muscles. It simply means concentrating on parts of the body in a certain way. Visualisation is a powerful tool when used with basic movements and breathing. A few of the techniques involve an imaginary aid such as the visualisation of a sandbag or a pulley or a heavy chain to weigh down a part of the body or encourage it to release in a certain direction. Some of these techniques can be used anywhere during a quiet moment without bringing any attention to yourself. It takes physical and mental activity to stay young and healthy, particularly in the structural sense, and we need to use a combination of both.

Breathing

All the techniques use and harness the potent influence of correct breathing. Few of us breathe properly and yet proper breathing on its own is a powerful healing process. Breathing alone can change structure. Just as habitually holding and restricting the breath can progressively tighten the body, conscious and directed breathing helps to release and change it both superficially and deeply. You can actually "feel" parts of your body broaden, lengthen, release, open and soften as you exhale. In all the techniques involving voluntary movement you should exaggerate the movement towards the end of each exhalation. Some instructions suggest "sighing" to enhance the effect of breathing out and sometimes it is suggested that you pull the belly back against the spine as you exhale to enhance and stabilise a given technique. Sometimes you are asked to breathe down through your heels. You imagine your exhalation moving down your body through your legs and heels into the floor. This helps to ground you through your legs and pelvis and free your spine, shoulders and head.

Don't take great big breaths, don't puff and blow, just breathe slowly, inhaling through the nose. Exhaling through the mouth should not become a habit while you are practising the techniques, as although it gives a quicker result in terms of releasing muscles, breathing out through the nose takes longer and gives more time to sense and visualise imagined movement. Ideally your belly should expand slightly as you inhale and retract or reduce in size as you exhale. You need to concentrate on correct breathing as much as on the techniques themselves, as it is an integral part of the process of changing structure.

Choices

The number of techniques given for each part of the body varies. This is because some parts of the structure need fewer techniques to free and balance them while others have the capacity for a much wider range of movements and positions. For example, there are eight techniques specifically for positioning the pelvis and five for centring the head, but more than thirty techniques for the hips and twenty for the spine. Some are repeated, e.g. some techniques for the knees are used again for the hips, but the focus is different.

The idea is not to go through all the techniques in one go, but to pick out your own routines or your own way of working from what's been given. To start you off suggested routines are provided at the end of the main sections (page 115).

You have a choice of approach.

- Work through only one part of the body at each session, alternating with routines that cover the whole body. Start with the feet and work up; or
- Stick to the suggested routines that cover the whole body and occasionally put

emphasis on the area or areas where you feel especially tight or restricted; or

- If you are familiar with body work, work out your own routines.

The important thing is to cover the whole body in one way or another and make progress.

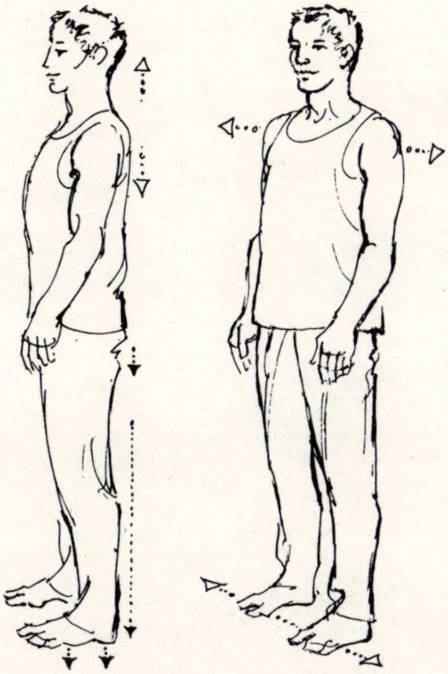

The Standing and Lying Release Positions

Many of the sections, techniques and routines start and/or end with what is called the standing release position (SRP) and the lying release position (LRP). The SRP is particularly useful as you can "slip" into it any time, anywhere in order to "release" on the spot.

The Standing Release Position

Stand with your feet roughly 20 cm apart and almost parallel. Your big toes should be slightly closer to each other than your heels. Spread your toes. Take 6 slightly deeper breaths and feel the following each time you *exhale.*

- Weight through your heels, the outer edge of your feet and the base of your big toes.
- Your tail bone dropping.
- Heavy wrists and elbows.
- The back of your shoulders widening and your neck lengthening upwards.

The Lying Release Position

Lie on your back, knees bent, feet a small distance apart and in line with the knees and hips.

- Tuck your chin in slightly to lengthen the back of your neck. If your neck tends to arch place a small pillow or folded towel under your head.
- Cross your arms over the front of your chest as loosely as possible.
- Some people will need to have their knees slightly closer together than their feet to counteract the tendency for the knees to fall apart.
- Each time you exhale feel your pelvis and lower back sink into the floor, the space between your shoulder blades widen, the back of your neck settle towards the floor and the space between your ears at the back of your head broadening.

Practise this for at least 10 to 15 exhalations.

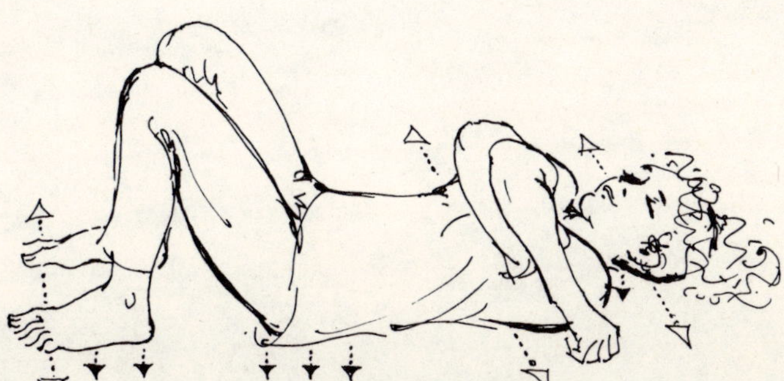

The Lower Structure

The Feet

There is probably no part of the human structure more abused, misused or underestimated in its influence on the entire body than the foot. We do all kinds of things to our feet that inhibit them and their ability to work well. The feet of some of the most health-conscious people leave much to be desired. Many people arrive for their first session wearing training shoes expecting to keep them on. When the shoes come off it is amazing to see feet in such poor condition. We lock our feet into often unsuitable footwear. Even in summer many people rarely expose their feet or employ techniques that attend to their needs. Yet our feet form our very foundations.

Feet have two functions, to support the body above them and to act as shock-absorbers. They need strength to support weight and elasticity to prevent jarring. A rigid foot is a poor supporter and an even poorer shock-absorber. Each foot has 26 bones and 32 joints, so we actually stand, walk and run on 64 joints. This number of joints should be able to provide a variety of twisting movements that allow us to adapt to uneven surfaces or to turn suddenly when running. Both stability and elasticity are provided by the three arches of each foot: an inner arch, the one that most people are familiar with; an outer arch which few people are aware of because the foot appears so flat in this area; and an arch that runs across the front of the foot. The arches are stabilised by very strong muscles too large to be contained in the feet themselves and they operate from the lower leg (shin and calf muscles) via strong tendons extending down into the feet. The shock-absorbing function of the arches is essential for the flexibility and spring of gait. Any condition that flattens, exaggerates or interferes with the arches can seriously interfere with body mechanics as a whole.

Flat Feet

We are all born with flat feet. The arches start to form shortly after birth, at first by the clasping motion all babies make with their feet, and subsequently by the muscular work of the lower legs in crawling, standing and walking. If the arch fails to form, this is congenital flat foot, but it is rare. The majority of flat feet respond to exercise. Many people with flattish feet get no pain or discomfort in the feet themselves, but strain tends to build higher up, in the knees, pelvis, lower back and spine as a whole. This eventually disturbs general ease and freedom of movement, drains vital energy and may lead to fatigue and other symptoms.

Hollow Foot

A high exaggerated arch is common, but less so than flat foot. The foot is usually very rigid, which may lead to painful arthritis between the bones of the foot. Hollow foot also has repercussions further up the structure and causes structural strain and fatigue.

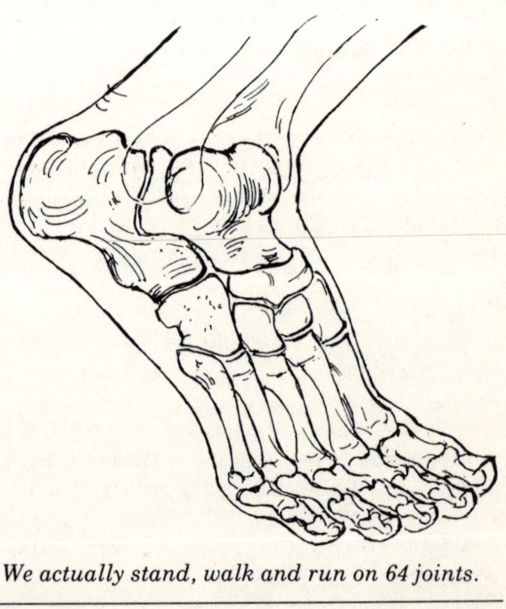

We actually stand, walk and run on 64 joints.

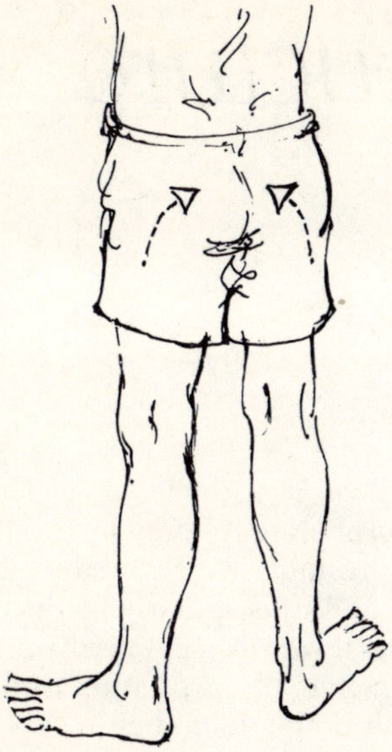

Toeing out closes the pelvic joints and puts strain on the lower back.

Toeing Out
This means both feet turning out. The common problem when both big toes veer out is not the same thing and is usually related to flat feet and fallen arches. Turned out feet are common in dancers due to their training, but most people show varying degrees of "turned-outness" when they stand, and very few automatically and spontaneously walk with the feet parallel. With chronically toed-out feet, the forward and backward movement of the ankle and knee is disturbed. They stiffen and this changes the line of force through the hips which closes and stiffens joints at the back of the pelvis and puts strain on the lower back.

Toeing In
Toeing in is the reverse of toeing out. Forces through the hips are also altered, subsequently overstretching the pelvic joints and putting strain on the lower back.

Toes
Perfect toes are rare and nearly everyone has some degree of stiffness and deformity in the toes. Few people can spread, flex or extend their toes fully and yet they too have a role to play in the balance of the body. Stiff and cramped toes not only affect general structural balance but also retain trapped energy that would be better off circulating through the rest of the body.

Whether you have a classifiable foot imbalance or not, the point is that the majority of people have some degree of structural disturbance between the bones of their feet. This affects the foot's ability to absorb shock, support weight and adjust effectively to uneven surfaces, and this may set up strain through the entire structure. However, problems higher up in the body may also affect the foot. Foot imbalances often result from imbalances in the lower leg muscles, and hip imbalances can just as easily reflect down to the foot as the other way round.

Freeing the Feet
All these techniques collectively assist in freeing and balancing the feet and attending to all their common imbalances.

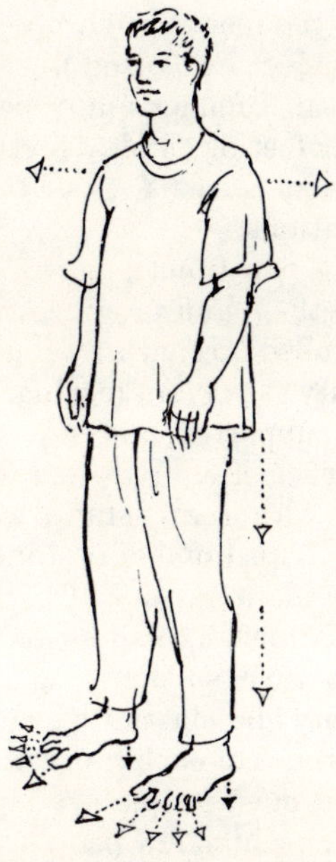

Feet 1
From the standing release position (SRP) spread your toes as wide apart as you can. It is particularly important to cultivate the ability to separate the big toe from the second toe. This takes practice but eventually you should achieve a wide and even spread.

Practise this for at least 6 breaths sensing the imprint of your feet as you exhale.

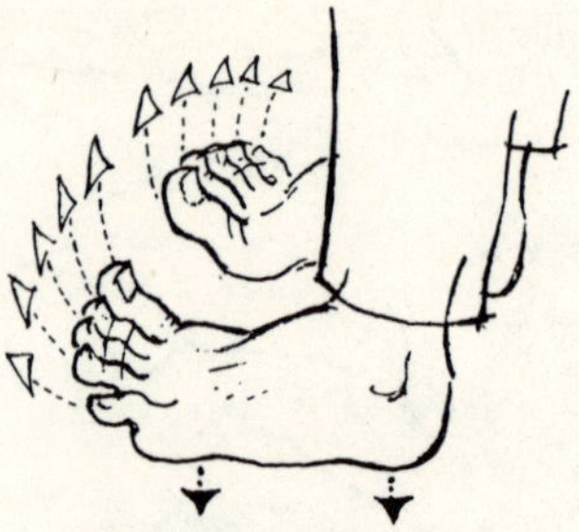

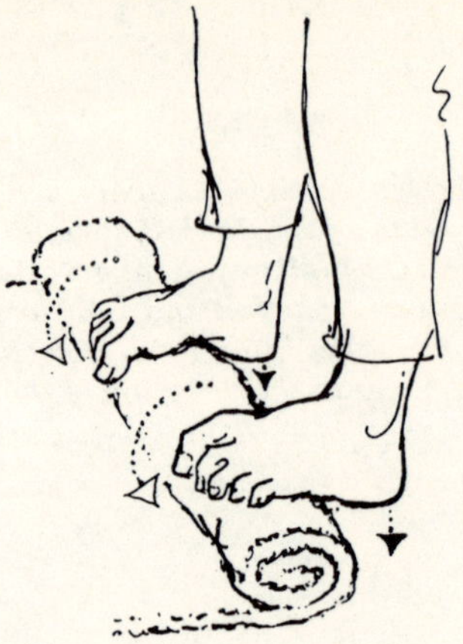

Feet 2
From the SRP spread your toes and lift them as high as you can, keeping the balls of your feet on the floor. This raises the arches.
Practise for 6 breaths, exhaling down through your heels and the balls of your feet.

Feet 3
From the SRP place a rolled towel under your feet, keeping your heels on the floor.
Grip the towel firmly with your feet by curling your toes. Practise this for at least 6 breaths, always exhaling down through your heels.

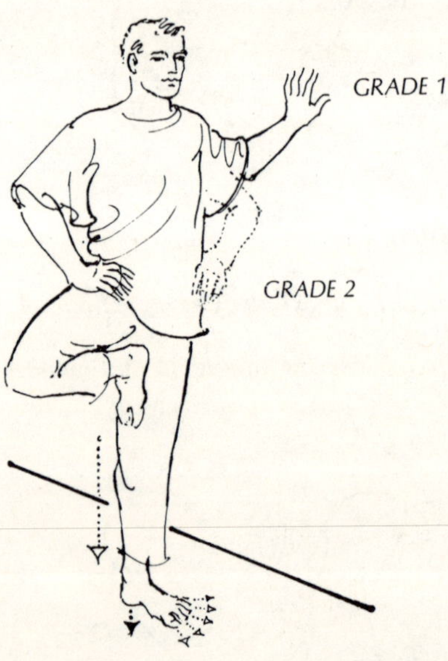

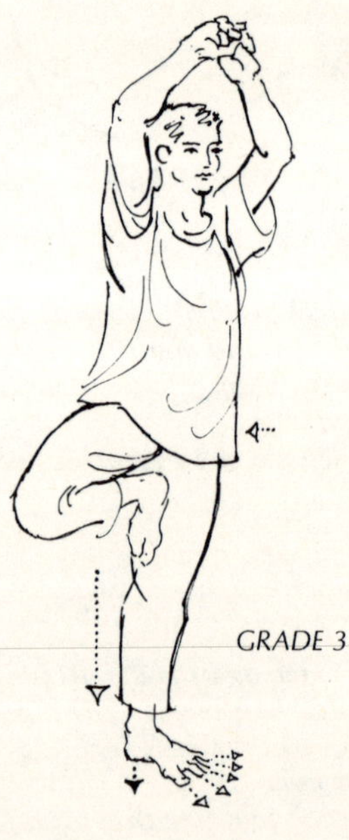

Feet 4
From the SRP pull up one heel on to your opposite thigh as high as possible. Use one hand on a wall to balance if you need to (Grade 1). Spread the toes of the standing foot wide, exhaling down through the heel. Feel the foot working.
Practise for at least 6 breaths and then change sides. When you can balance easily try Grade 2 and then Grade 3, keeping the shoulders soft and a sense of the tail bone dropping down towards your standing heel.

Feet 5

With your feet a few centimetres apart, squat down holding on to a table or desk to balance and lift your heels as high as you can by bending at the joints between your feet and your toes.

Practise for 6 breaths lifting and projecting your heels and knees in the direction of the arrows.

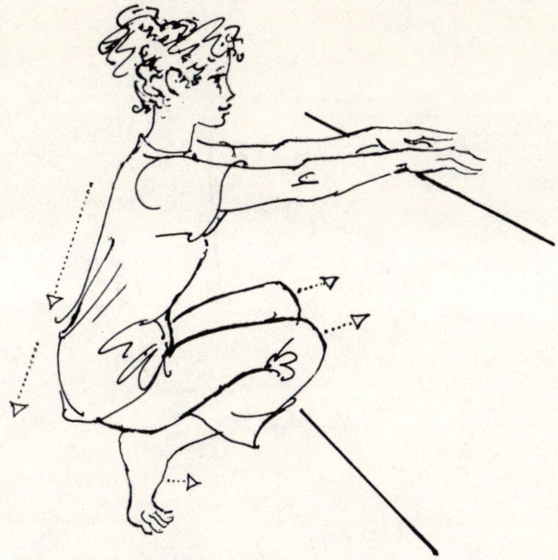

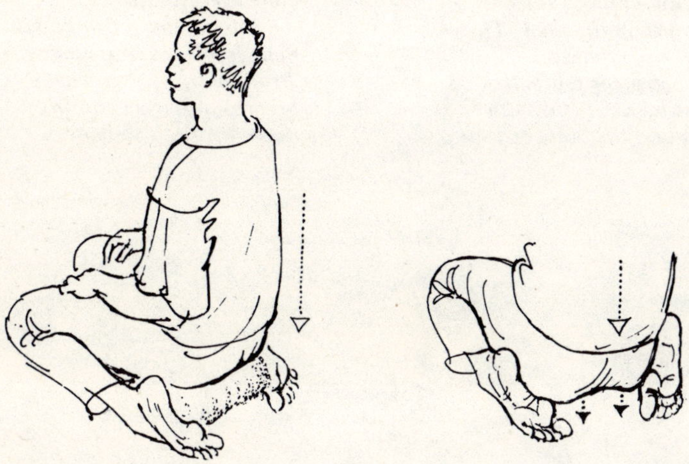

Feet 6

Sit between your feet and roll your calves outwards with your hands. Your big toes should point towards each other behind you.

Let your pelvis sink down to the floor and feel heavy as you exhale. Use a cushion to alleviate any initial discomfort.

Practise for at least 8 to 12 breaths, keeping very relaxed in the shoulders and long in the neck.

Feet 7

Sitting with your back against a wall twist each foot in a "wringing" movement working down its entire length. And then pull each toe backward and forward.

You can work each foot like this for a few minutes. Don't be scared of working hard at these techniques.

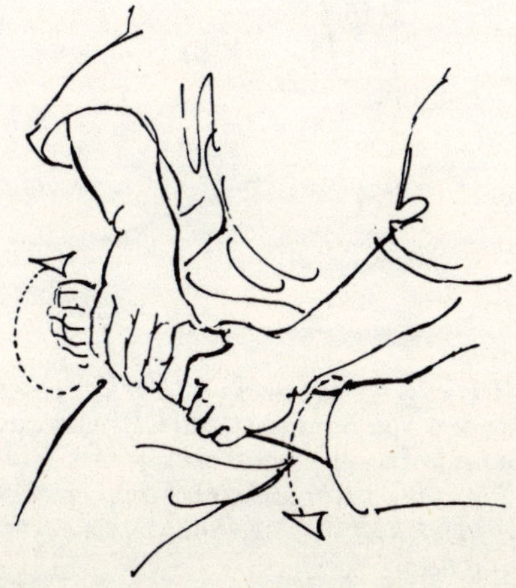

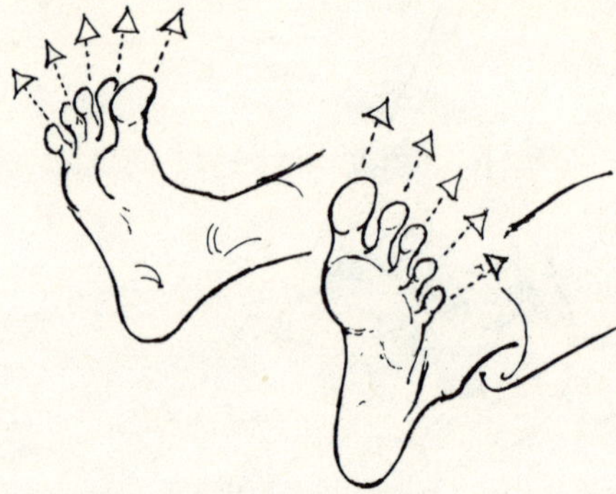

Feet 8
Sitting on the floor spread your toes strongly.
Practise for at least 6 breaths.
Your feet may ache slightly as you do this, which shows that the necessary muscles are working.

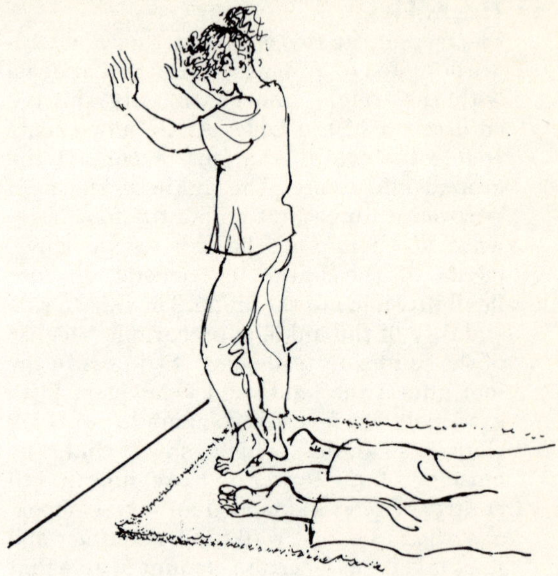

Feet 9
Another person can massage your feet with his or her heels. This is a powerful technique for loosening all the joints of the feet. Work on a blanket for comfort.
The person working rubs his or her heels together and performs a kind of mini-walk all over your soles. Obviously the pressure must be graded to suit each individual's tolerance.
A minute or two on each foot should be sufficient.

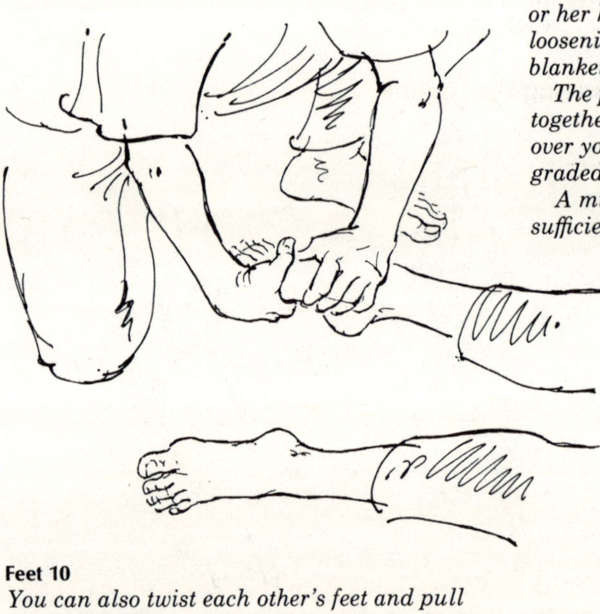

Feet 10
You can also twist each other's feet and pull and bend the toes. It is important to fix the foot with one hand while twisting an adjoining part with the other.
In all these assisted techniques, remember to grade your approach to suit the other person's tolerance. Stop if it hurts.

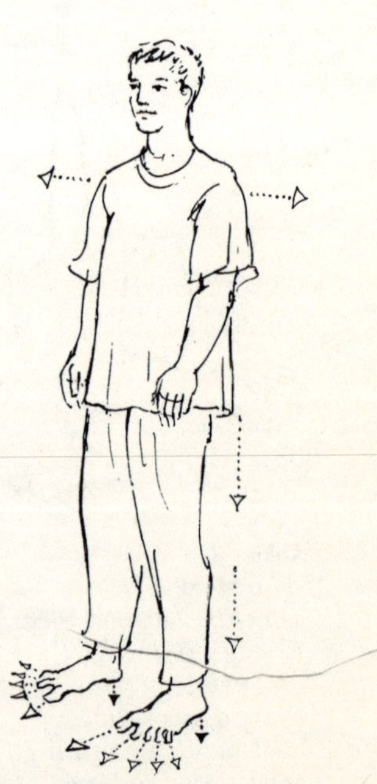

Feet 11
In the SRP, spread the toes again and feel the general difference in your feet compared to when you first started.

The Ankles

The feet and ankles work together and both are designed to form a mechanism that deals with the weight and continually shifting adjustment of the body. Ankle movements enable the sole of the foot to contact the ground effectively. The ankle works as a horizontal hinge that points the foot backward and forward. The side-to-side movements of the lower leg depend on foot flexibility and not the ankle. The side-to-side stability of the ankle is precarious because of the joint's natural shape. Stiffness in the foot affects the ankle and vice versa. With extremely flat feet it is common to see thick shapeless ankles which show that the muscles of the lower leg are not in full control. The ankle is also an active shock-absorber during walking, running and jumping; it has a certain amount of give that lessens the impact transmitted upward into the spine. The ankle's many sensory nerve-endings give it the awareness that is vital in correcting us when we are off balance.

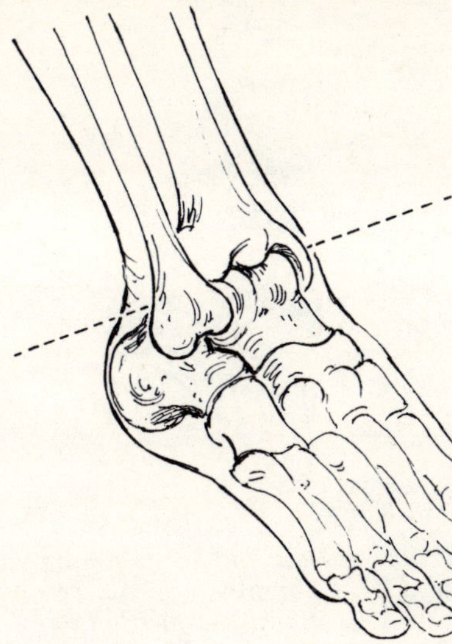

The ankle works as a horizontal hinge

Balancing the Ankles

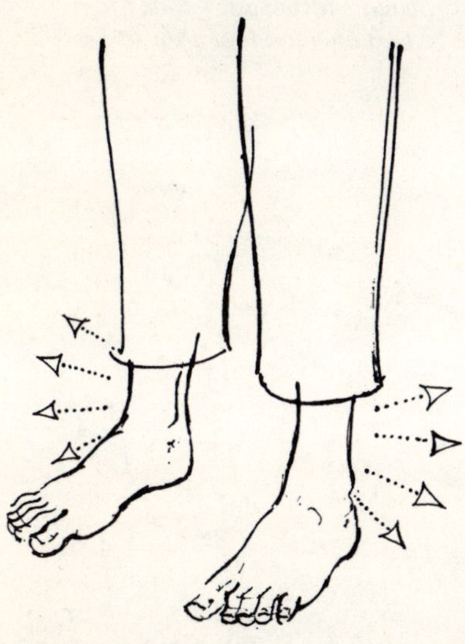

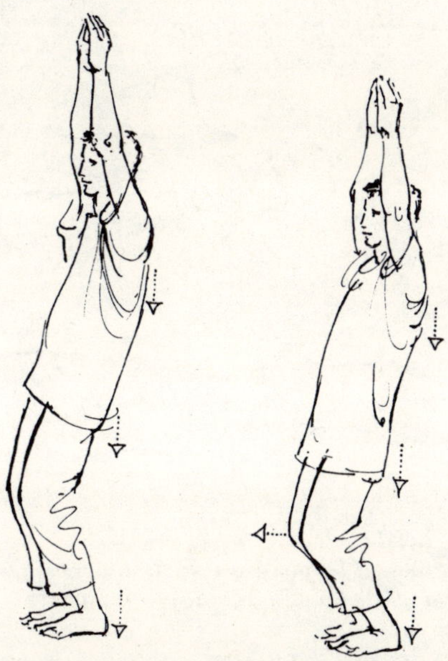

Ankles 1

As a start it is sometimes a good idea to stand in the SRP and exhale a few times down into your heels while imagining or visualising inner space inside your ankles.

Ankles 2

With your feet and knees together stretch your arms upwards with your palms and fingers together.

Slowly project your knees forward as far as you can while keeping your heels on the floor.

The idea is to sink your pelvis as low as possible without arching your back.

Practise for at least 6 breaths and only sink lower on each exhalation.

Remember the arrows depict lines of movement.

Ankles 3

Stand with your legs wide apart and your toes turned slightly inwards.

As you exhale slowly bring the trunk forward, pushing the outside of your feet firmly into the floor.

Keep your weight through your heels to keep your pelvis centred over your ankles.

Completely release between the shoulder blades.

In Grade 3 feel your spine lengthen down towards the floor.

Practise for 6 breaths and come up slowly, exhaling.

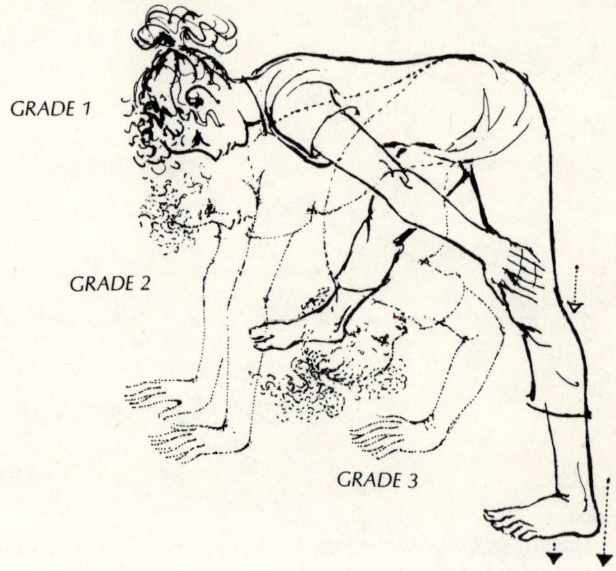

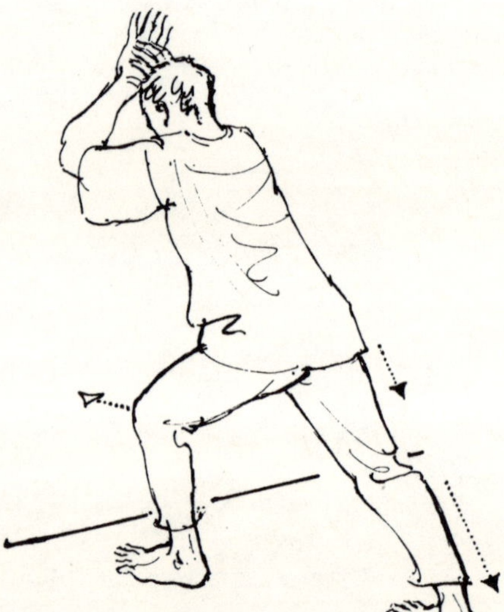

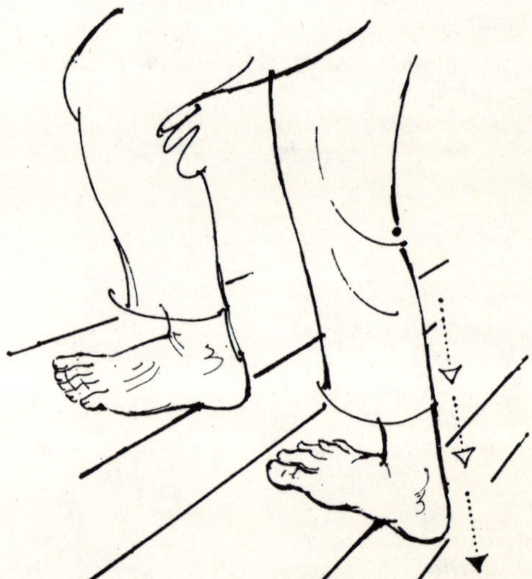

Ankles 4

In this position you can easily and strongly stretch the back of your back calf and ankle.

Turn your back foot inwards, toes pointing towards the wall.

Push your back heel down as you exhale.

Remember consciously to release the area being stretched.

Increasing the bend of the front knee exaggerates the stretch if necessary.

Keep released between the shoulder blades and don't tense up your shoulders or neck.

Practise for 6 breaths and change sides.

Ankles 5

With one foot halfway off a step or a stair, allow your body weight to drop through the heel. Hold on to a wall or banister for balance.

Visualise the back of your ankle and calf "softening and lengthening" each time you exhale.

Practise for 5 or 6 breaths on each leg.

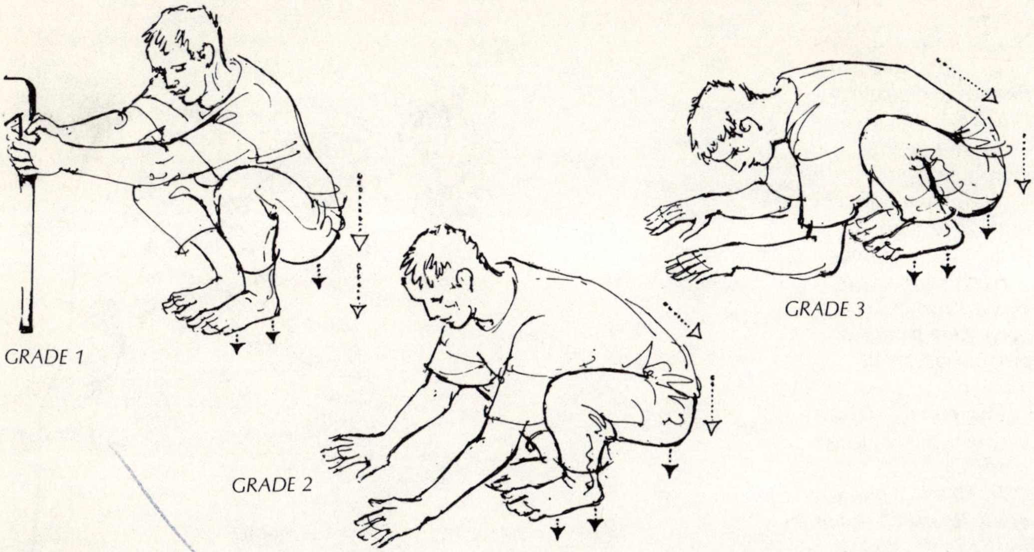

Ankles 6

With your feet and knees together squat down, keeping your heels on the floor. If your ankles are tight you will have to hold on to something to stop falling backwards.

Allow your knees to open slightly.

Each time you exhale visualise your tail bone dropping.

When Grade 2 is easy, try Grade 3 which involves dropping your trunk between your knees and sinking your elbows towards the floor during each exhalation.

Through all grades, release and relax the shoulders and between the shoulder blades as much as possible.

For some people achieving Grade 2 will probably be sufficient.

Practise for 8 breaths.

Ankles 7

Sit in position A.

Stretch forward as in B.

Spread your hands wide keeping them shoulder width and push up into position C.

Release the chest.

Lengthen the lower back and push the heels down towards the end of each exhalation.

Imagine the skin at the back of the knees and calves softening each time you exhale.

Practise for 6 breaths.

N.B. Arrange a folded blanket underneath the heels if the calf sensation is too intense to begin with.

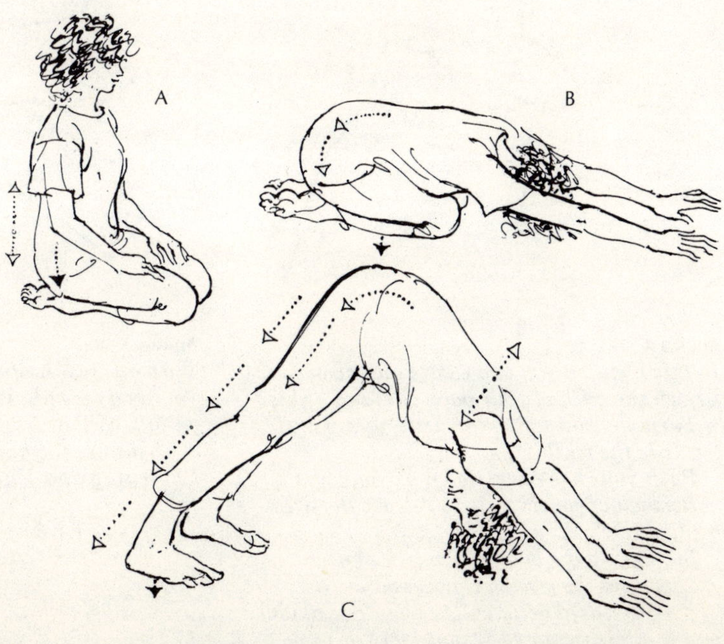

Ankles 8

For stiff ankles simply sit on your heels (Grade 1).

Roll your calves outwards and widen your feet to allow your buttocks to sink towards the floor.

Use a cushion to ease unnecessary discomfort especially in the knees (Grade 2).

When this is comfortable, try it without a cushion (Grade 3).

Tie your ankles together and sit on your heels as in Grade 4—this gives a very strong stretch at the front of the feet and ankles but is ideal for balancing the foot on the leg at the ankle joint itself.

In all grades pay attention to your breathing. Visualise the back of your pelvis dropping and the area of stretch softening each time you exhale.

Practise for at least 8 breaths.

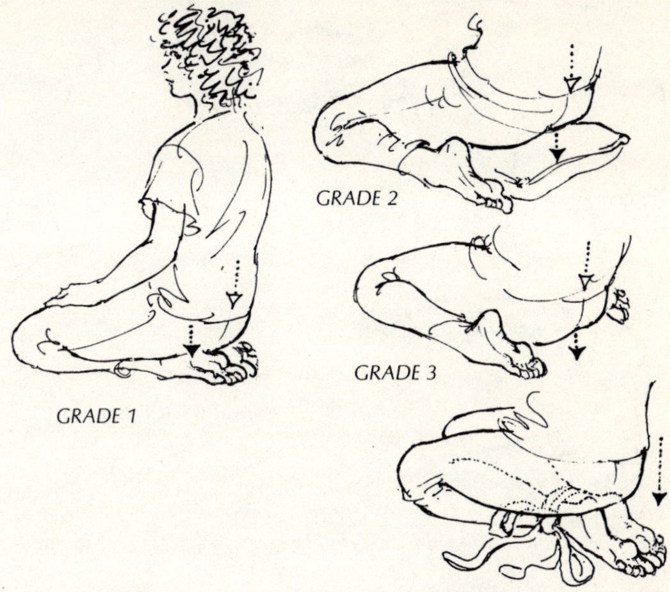

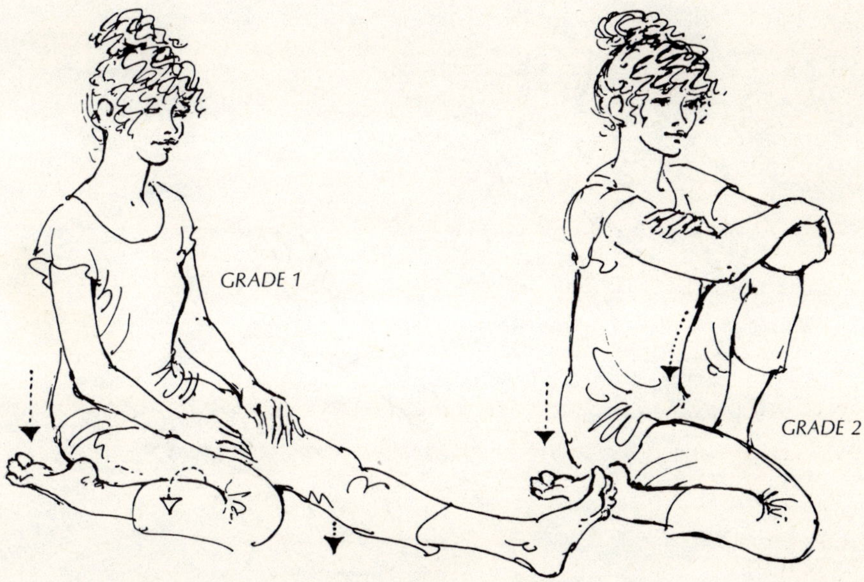

Ankles 9

If Grade 3 of Ankles 8 was easy, try this technique.

Sit between your feet and straighten out one leg.

Roll out the calf of the bent leg with one hand and ease your buttocks to the floor.

Support yourself with your hand if you are lopsided.

Each time you exhale imagine the pelvis dropping and becoming heavy and visualise the front of your foot and ankle softening.

Grade 2 involves bending up the straight leg and trying to exhale, keeping both buttocks to the floor with equal pressure.

Practise either or both techniques for at least 6 breaths on each side.

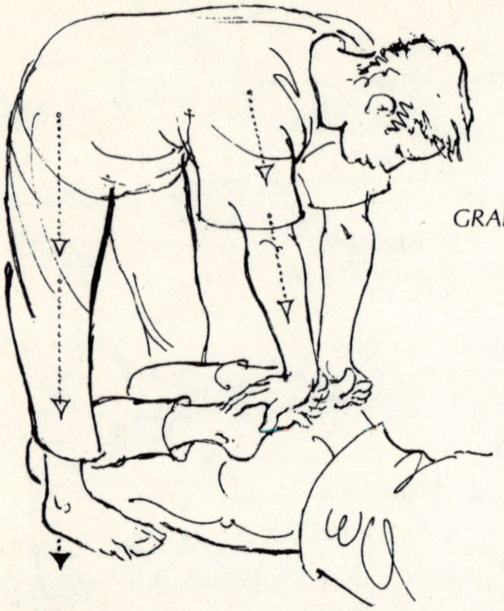

GRADE 1

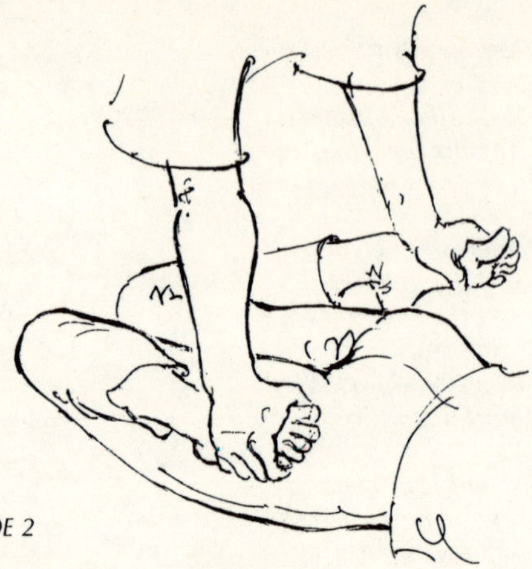

GRADE 2

Ankles 10

Lie face down while someone slowly stretches your feet towards your buttocks, clasping your feet beneath the toes.

The person helping should exaggerate the movement towards the end of your exhalations until your heels touch your buttocks (Grade 1).

If this was easy, Grade 2 involves widening the heels and easing them down on either side of your hips.

The person helping can use his or her own feet to stop your knees sliding too far apart.

Practise for 6 breaths.

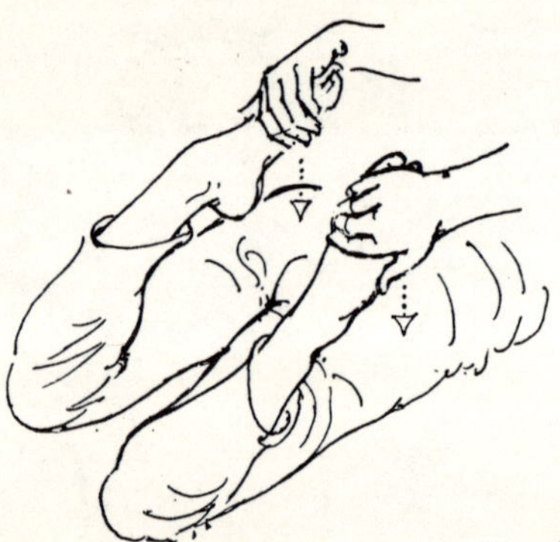

GRADE 1

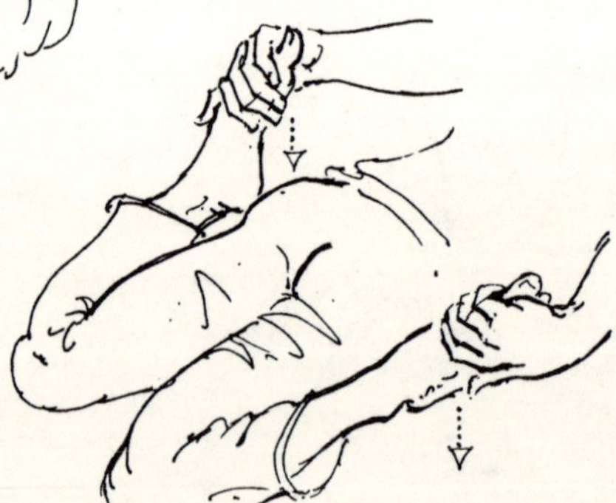

GRADE 2

Ankles 11

If you feel ready, practise Ankles 10 by yourself.

With knees slightly apart, pull your feet downwards towards the end of each exhalation.

As in the previous technique, if your heels touch your buttocks easily, ease your feet down towards the outsides of your hips.

Remember you need a certain amount of resistance to "bite on" in order consciously to release and soften the area where you feel the most tension. In this case it may be the front of your thighs, your knees, or the front of your feet or ankles.

Practise for at least 4 breaths.

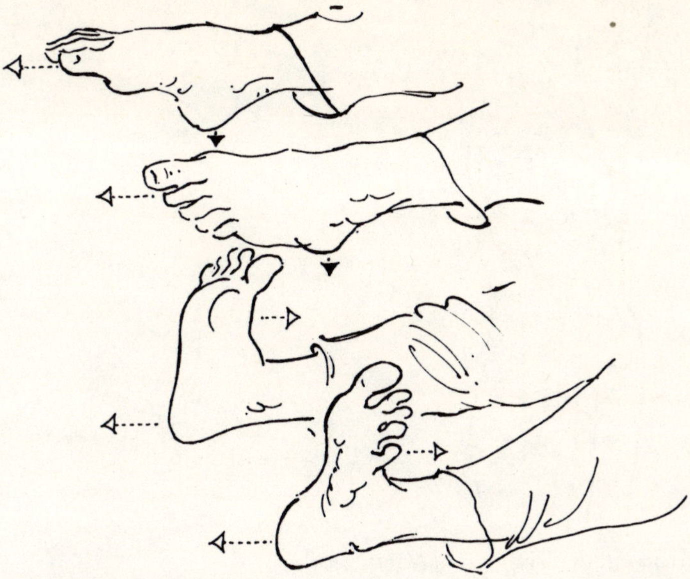

Ankles 12
Simply lie on your back strongly pointing your toes away from you for 4 breaths and then strongly drawing them back towards your knees for 4 breaths.

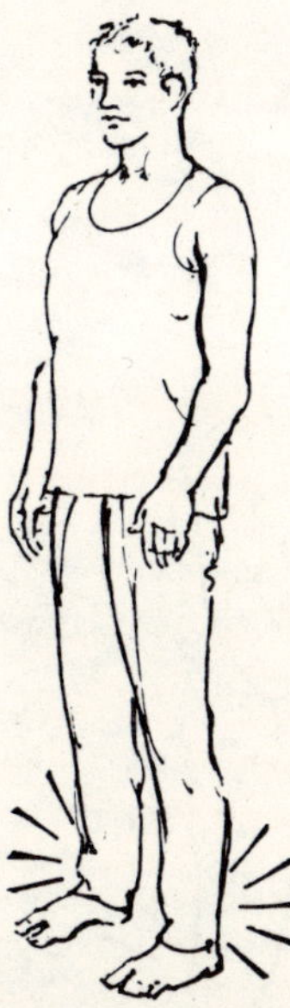

Ankles 13
To finish the ankle techniques stand in the SRP and once more visualise inner space in your ankles.

They should feel more alive, softer and your sense of them should be generally more defined.

The Knees

The knee is the largest joint in the body. Like the ankle, it is a horizontal hinge allowing it to bend and straighten, but it also turns and twists slightly when bent. The structure of the knee has two effects. Firstly, its strong binding ligaments and its strong protective muscles give it great stability, essential for it to transfer the entire body weight through the long bones of the leg from the pelvis to the foot. Secondly, it has wide freedom of movement because the bones are not closely bound within their own configuration. The knee is most stable when straight, but sacrifices stability for the great mobility needed for running, climbing and jumping etc, and so that it can effectively accommodate itself to the changes in the foot caused by irregularities of the ground. Ideally, movement of the knee and ankle should be parallel, the joints centred one above the other. The knee is the most vulnerable part of the leg. Accidents and injuries are common to the knee but its most frequent *underlying* problem, like most other joints, is an exaggerated force of compression. Muscles influencing the knee easily shorten, tending to compress and even twist the joint, making it unstable and functionally stiff. Such a knee is a poor shock-absorber and its lack of resilience leaves it wide open to all kinds of strain, injury and wear-and-tear arthritis. Any unnatural stiffening of the knee upsets the transfer of body weight and the balance of the structure as a whole.

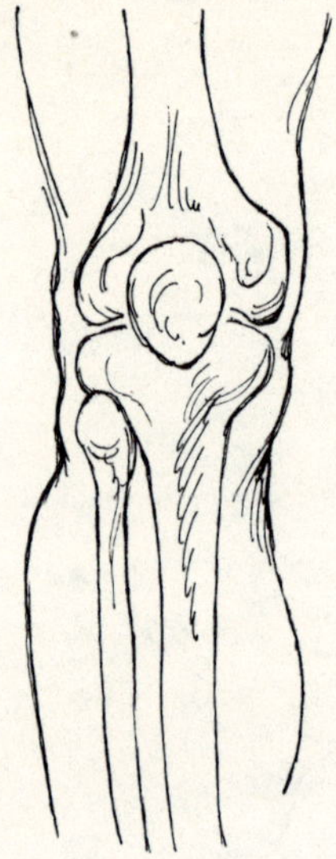

The most frequent underlying *problem in the knee is an exaggerated force of compression.*

Opening the Knees

The knees are vulnerable and demand a particularly slow and easy approach. By all means tolerate a strong stretching sensation in the knees but sharp pain indicates that you are exceeding your present limitation. Remember that the subtleties are as important and in some cases even more so than the gross movements and positions. Some people can take months and even years to free, open, soften and balance the structure of their knee joints completely. However, each stage of progress and each little breakthrough provides its own benefits.

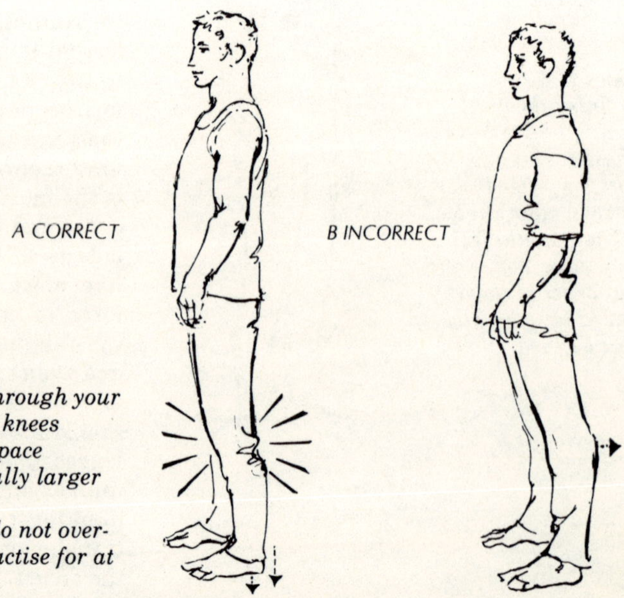

Knees 1

From the SRP and exhaling down through your heels, imagine the skin behind your knees softening and spreading, an inner space "inside" the knees becoming gradually larger each time you exhale.

N.B. Keep your knees straight but do not overextend them backwards as in B. Practise for at least 8 breaths.

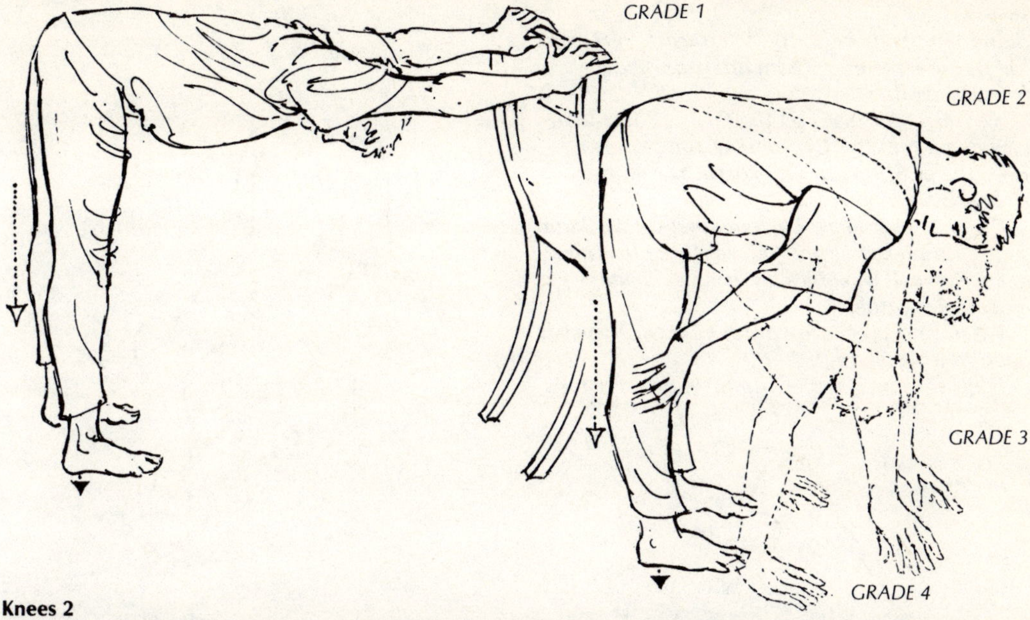

Knees 2

From the SRP bend at the hips and place your hands on a table or chair to form a right angle between your trunks and legs. You can use a mirror to check your position.
Relax between your shoulder blades.
Project your tail bone downwards to an imaginary spot between your heels.
Increase the forward bending gradually towards the end of your exhalations.
Each time you exhale imagine the skin behind your knees spreading and softening.
Work through the grades according to your own limitations. Excessive pain behind the knees indicates you are going too far too quickly.
Don't tolerate pain in the back under any circumstances.
Release, lengthen and soften for at least 6 exhalations.
N.B. *If maintaining a straight spine in Grade 1 is difficult, place your hands on something a little higher to widen the angle between your trunk and your legs.*

Knees 3

Stand with your feet roughly a metre apart, toes turned slightly in.

Turn your right foot completely out on its heel and bend your right knee slowly in stages until it lines up vertically above your ankle.

Each time you exhale lengthen your neck.

Drop and release your shoulders.

Allow your tail bone to drop slightly.

Practise for at least 4 breaths and then change sides.

This technique strengthens the bent knee while stretching the back of the straight knee.

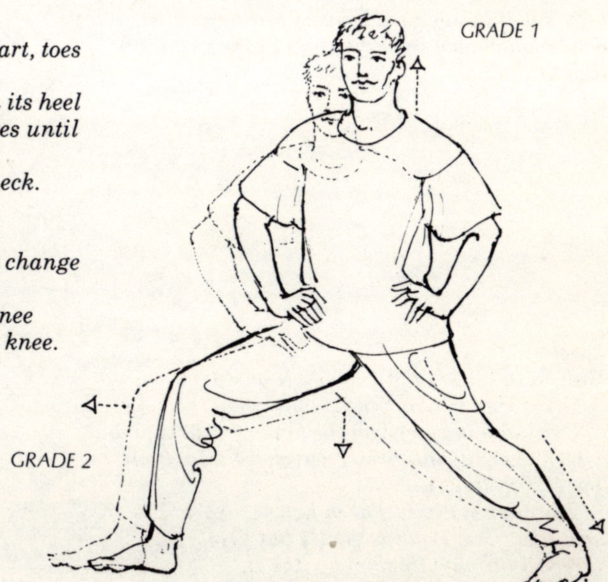

Knees 4

Stand with your back against a wall, with your feet parallel roughly 15 cm apart and 30 cm from the wall.

Keeping your heels on the floor, slide a little way down the wall by bending your knees. Hold the position for 4 to 6 breaths and then slide a little further.

Keeping your lower back against the wall and your chin tucked slightly in continue to slide down the wall in stages, holding each stage for at least 6 breaths.

When your thighs are parallel to the floor you have gone far enough.

Come up slowly, exhaling through your feet.

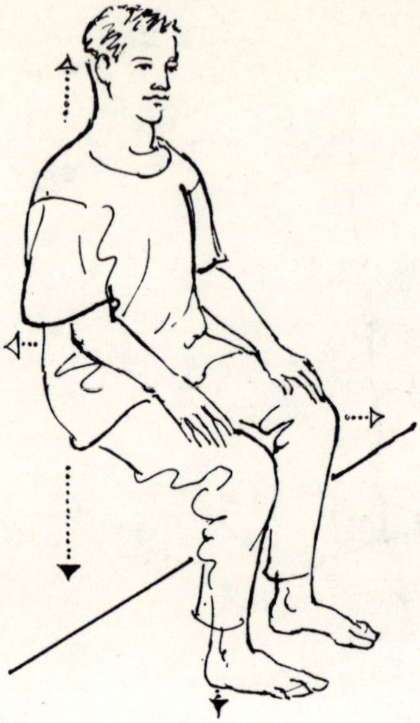

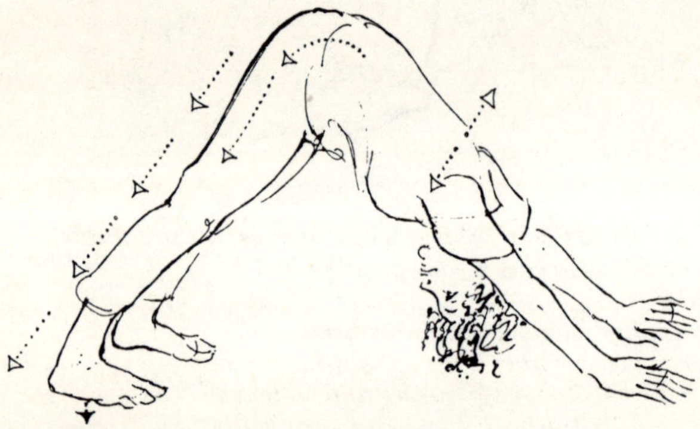

Knees 5

This technique is the same as Ankles 7.

The instruction is the same except *visualise in this case the skin at the back of your knees softening and spreading.*

Practise for at least 6 breaths, remembering to follow the suggested lines of projected movement shown by the arrows in the illustrations.

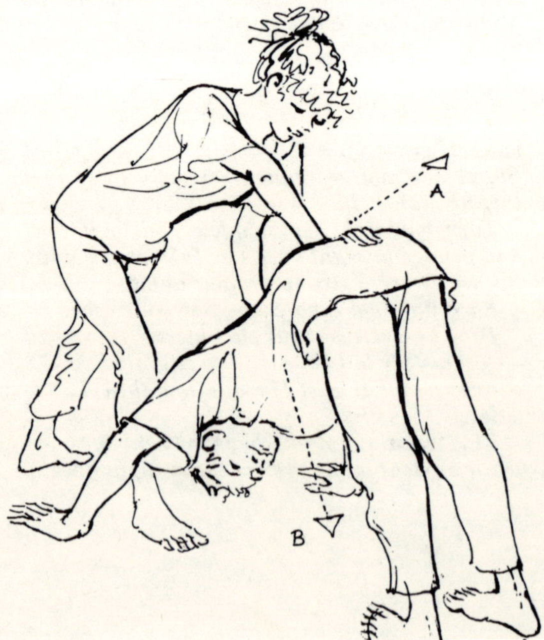

Knees 6

This technique is the same as Knees 5 but uses assistance from another person.

One hand is placed on the back of your pelvis which is gently but firmly directed through an imaginary line A.

The other hand is placed between your shoulder blades and is gently but firmly directed through imaginary line B.

Work and release for 4 to 6 breaths.

GRADE 1 GRADE 2 GRADE 3

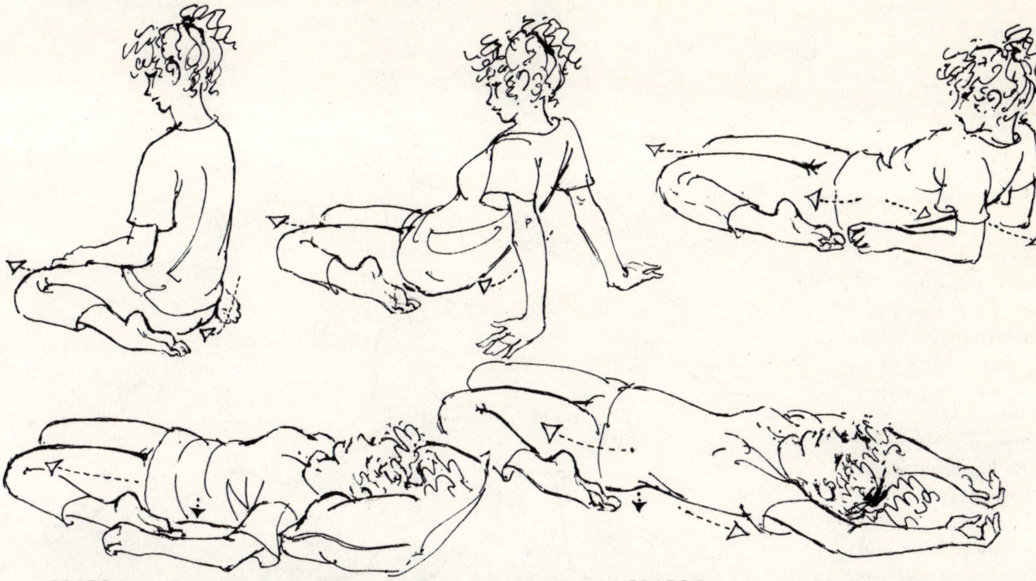

GRADE 4 GRADE 5

Knees 7

Sit on your heels as in Ankles 8.

Roll your calves out with your hands and ease your buttocks to the floor.

If this is difficult sit on a cushion.

Only move back as in Grade 2 when Grade 1 is comfortable with your buttocks on the floor.

It is especially important in this technique only to move on to the next grade when the previous one has become easier, and to resist the temptation to arch the lower back.

(That is why this technique necessitates 5 grades.)

Work, release and breathe for at least 6 breaths.

In each grade imagine a line of movement from your tail bone to between your knees.

Visualise your knees and the front of your thighs softening and spreading.

Each time you exhale, draw your belly back against your spine and allow your pelvis to sink and drop, also releasing the back of your ribs towards the floor and away from your pelvis.

Knees 8

This technique is the same as Knees 7 but another person may assist in all the grades from 1 to 5.

Weight is applied through the hip bones to help keep the pelvis tucked under and reduce the lower back curve.

The pelvis should be released slowly when finishing the technique to prevent the lower back suddenly "springing" into an exaggerated arch.

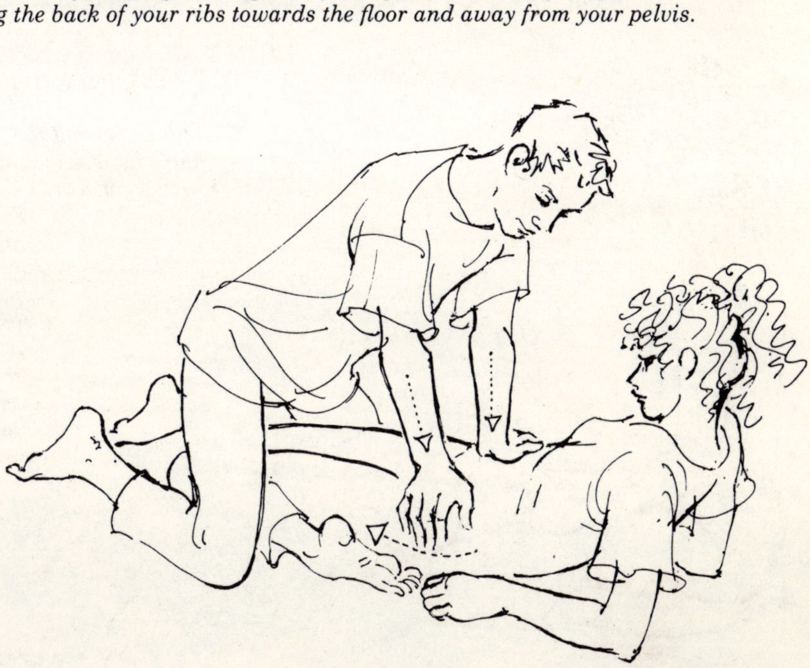

GRADE 1

GRADE 2

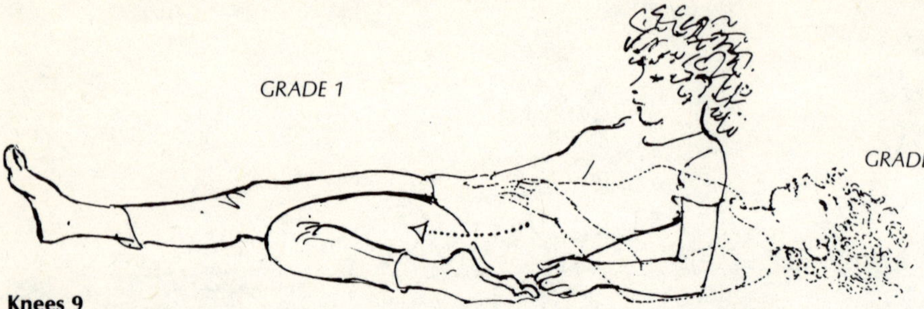

Knees 9

This technique is the same as Knees 7 but concentrates on one leg. Have your knees no more than 15 cm apart.

Again gradually work backwards from sitting to lying.

Imagine a line of movement from your tail bone to between your knees and visualise the skin of the bent knee and thigh softening and opening at the front.

ASSISTED

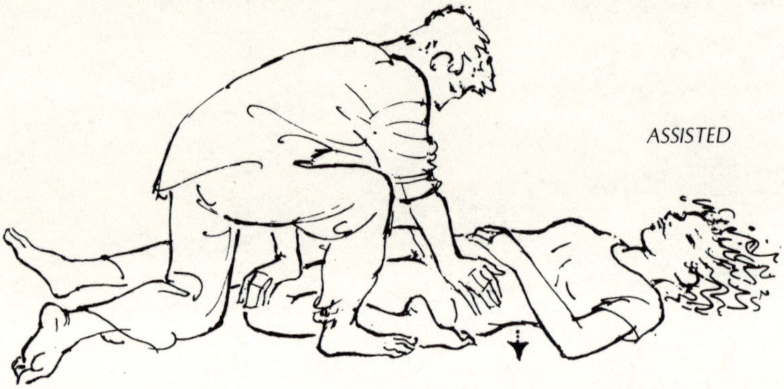

Allow your pelvis to sink, and resist the temptation to arch your lower back.

Someone may hold the hip and knee of the bent leg and gently lean in the direction of the arrows. He or she should apply more weight or pressure towards the end of your exhalations.

You can afford to be more adventurous in this technique and work and release for any number of breaths that feels comfortable.

Knees 10

This technique can exert a strong pull on the front of the knees, so ease into it very slowly.

Sit with your buttocks between your feet. Use a small cushion if your buttocks do not reach the floor.

Towards the end of each exhalation, slowly ease your hands forward without lifting your pelvis.

Don't go beyond the point where sensation in the knees becomes too strong.

Practise for 8 to 12 breaths.

The **subtle** *phase of this technique involves imagining your lower back lengthening and your tail bone sinking down between your heels.*

Imagine the front of your knees softening.

Release and relax your shoulders, upper back and neck.

If you can, try and release your whole body towards the end of each exhalation.

GRADE 1

GRADE 2

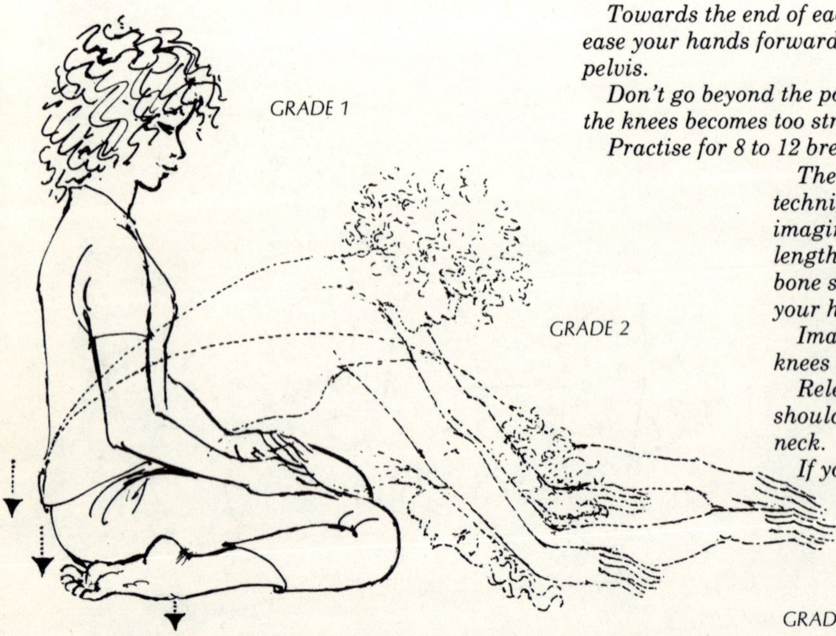

GRADE 3

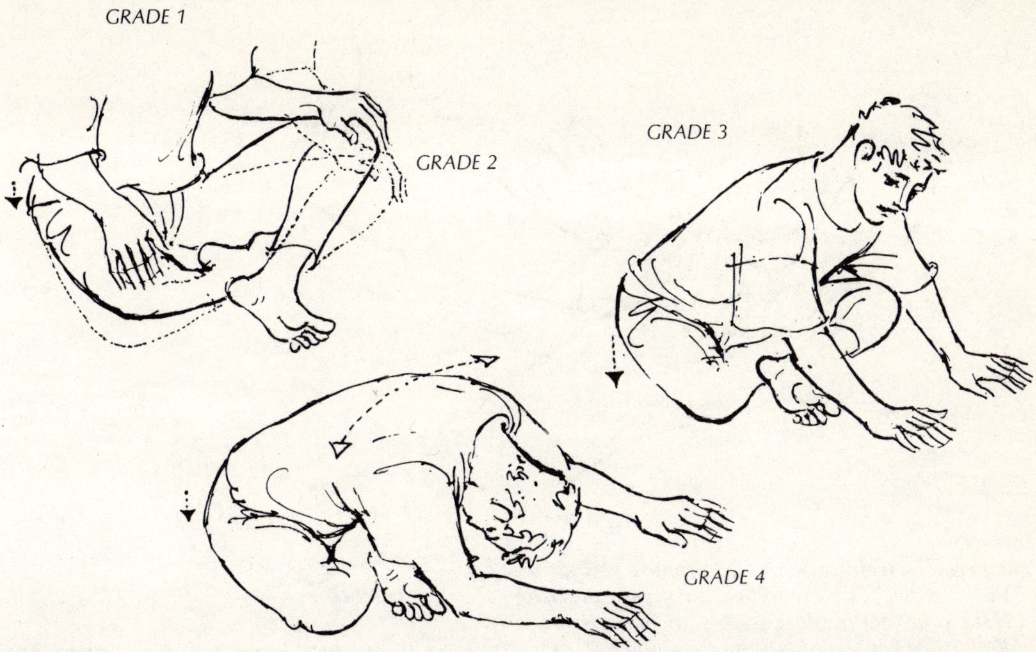

Knees 11

Sitting on the floor, pull both heels in towards your pubic bone, one heel directly in front of the other.

If your knees are a long way off the floor as in Grade 1, just rest your hands on your knees and allow your knees to drop slowly during each exhalation.

If Grade 2 is easy, slowly stretch forward keeping your tail bone down at the back.

The **subtle** *phase involves feeling very heavy in the pelvis, releasing the upper back and shoulders.*

If Grade 3 is easy, pull your belly back against your spine as you exhale to release you into Grade 4.

Practise for 8 to 10 slow breaths, then change your feet around and repeat.

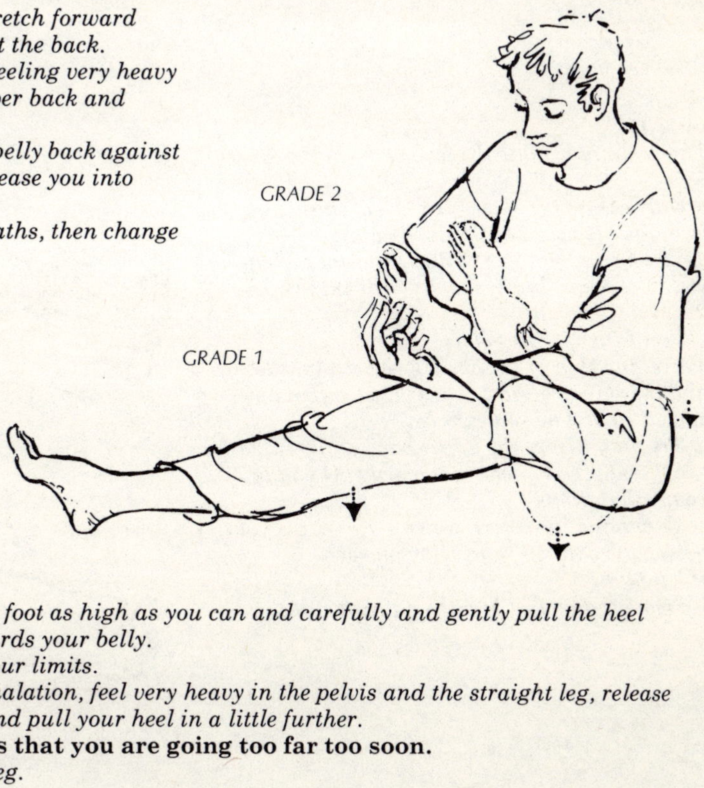

Knees 12

Slowly and carefully raise one foot as high as you can and carefully and gently pull the heel downwards and inwards towards your belly.

Do not force: work within your limits.

Towards the end of each exhalation, feel very heavy in the pelvis and the straight leg, release between the shoulder blades and pull your heel in a little further.

Pain in the knee indicates that you are going too far too soon.

Practise for 6 breaths each leg.

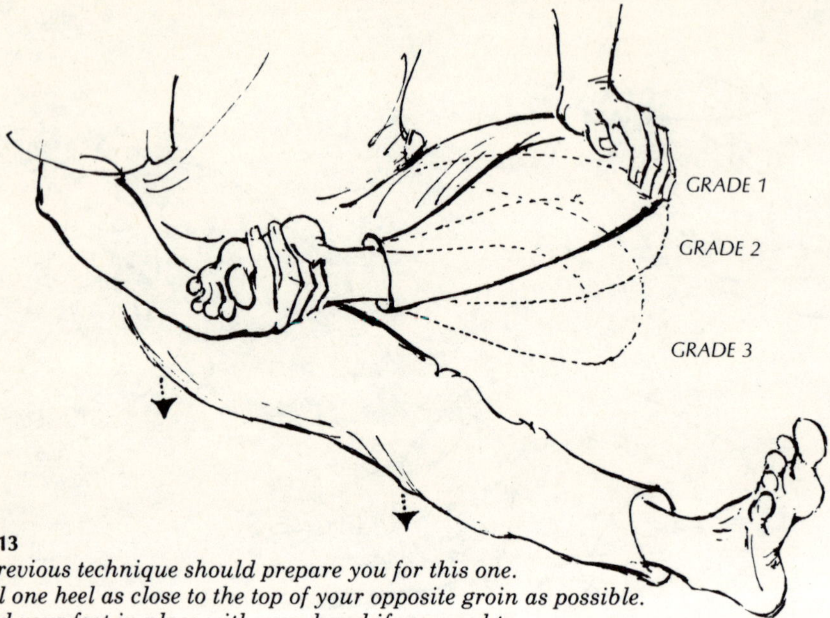

Knees 13

The previous technique should prepare you for this one.

Pull one heel as close to the top of your opposite groin as possible.

Hold your foot in place with your hand if you need to.

Each time you exhale allow the weight of your arm to help your bent knee gradually sink to the floor.

When Grade 2 is possible you will be able to start gently directing your bent knee inwards towards the straight leg as in Grade 3.

Each time you exhale feel heavy in the pelvis and try consciously to release any feeling of tension in the knee as much as possible.

Work for as many breaths as you feel appropriate.

No forcing.

Knees 14

This technique adds the forward bend to Knees 13.

Only attempt it when Grade 3 of that technique is possible.

You may need to use a strap at first to help you release gradually downwards into Grade 2.

Feel heavy in the pelvis.

Feel the skin at the back of the straight leg and the skin around the bent knee soften and spread each time you exhale.

Try and release the upper back and exaggerate the movement towards the end of your exhalations.

To enhance progress you can also draw your belly back against your spine on each exhalation.

No more than 6 to 8 breaths on each side.

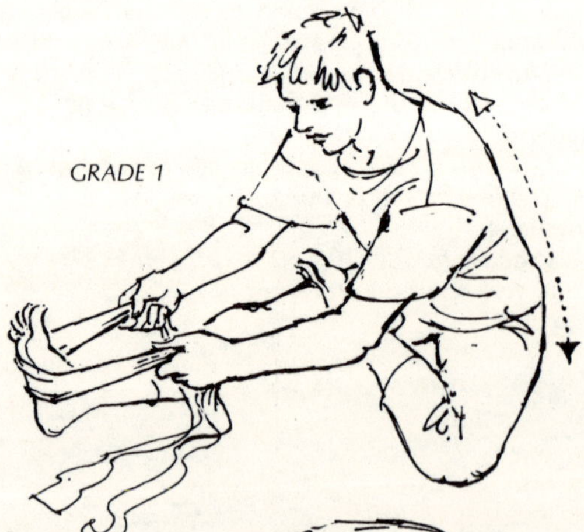

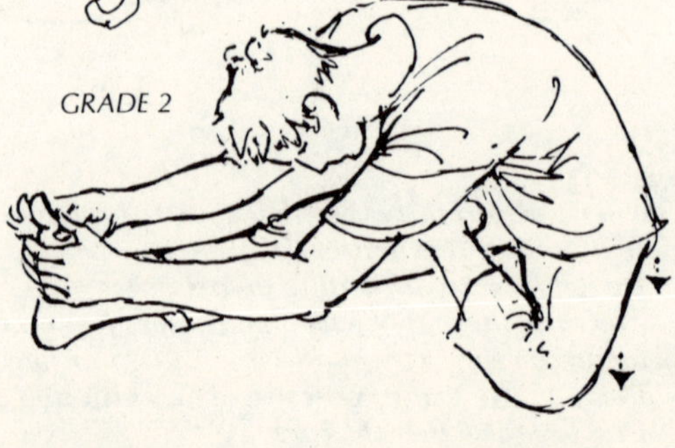

Knees 15

From Grade 2 or 3 of Knees 14 pull the foot of your straight leg underneath the thigh of your bent one.

Study the illustration for clarity.

Rest your hand on the upper knee and allow it to drop gradually as you exhale.

Each time you exhale, visualise the upper knee softening, relax the shoulders and let your arms go heavy.

Release for at least 8 breaths and then change sides.

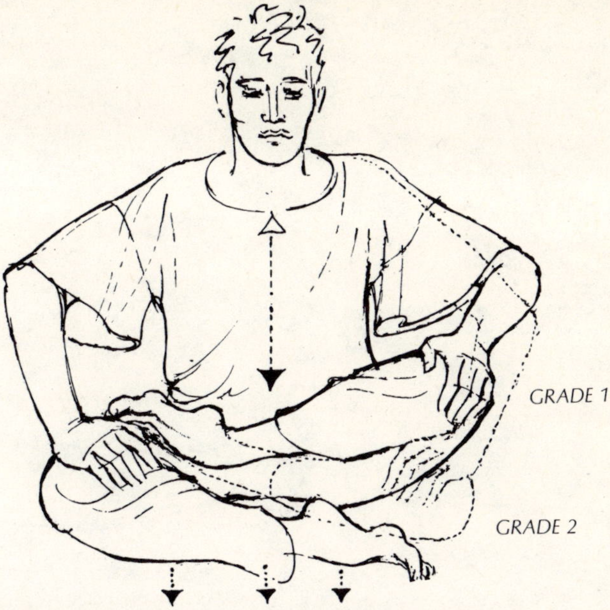

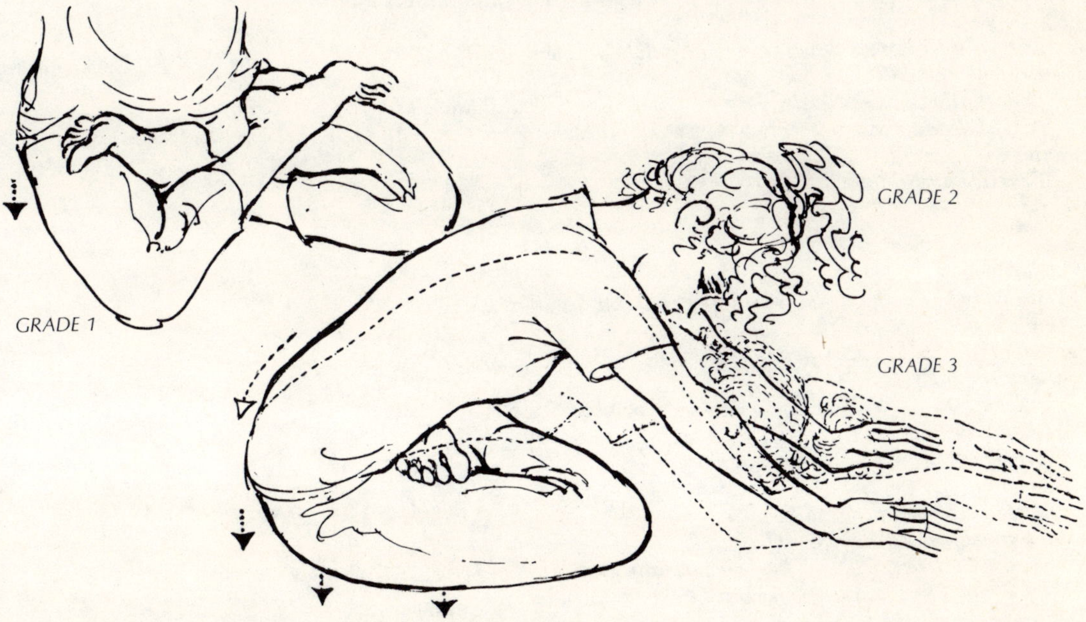

Knees 16

Many people have difficulty with this well-known yoga position, some even after years of practice.

It must not be forced.

It is not an essential technique but if the final grades of Knees 12, 13, 14 and 15 are relatively easy, it is well worth doing. It is simply a matter of placing first one and then the other heel well up on to the opposite thigh as close to the trunk as possible. It is usually easier to cross over one way than the other.

Try each way as in Grade 1.

Keep the pelvis feeling heavy each time you exhale and concentrate on lightening and releasing your spine and shoulders.

If this feels comfortable ease forward into Grade 2 or 3, leaving your pelvis behind you as a heavy stabilising force, so to speak.

Practise and release for at least 6 breaths.

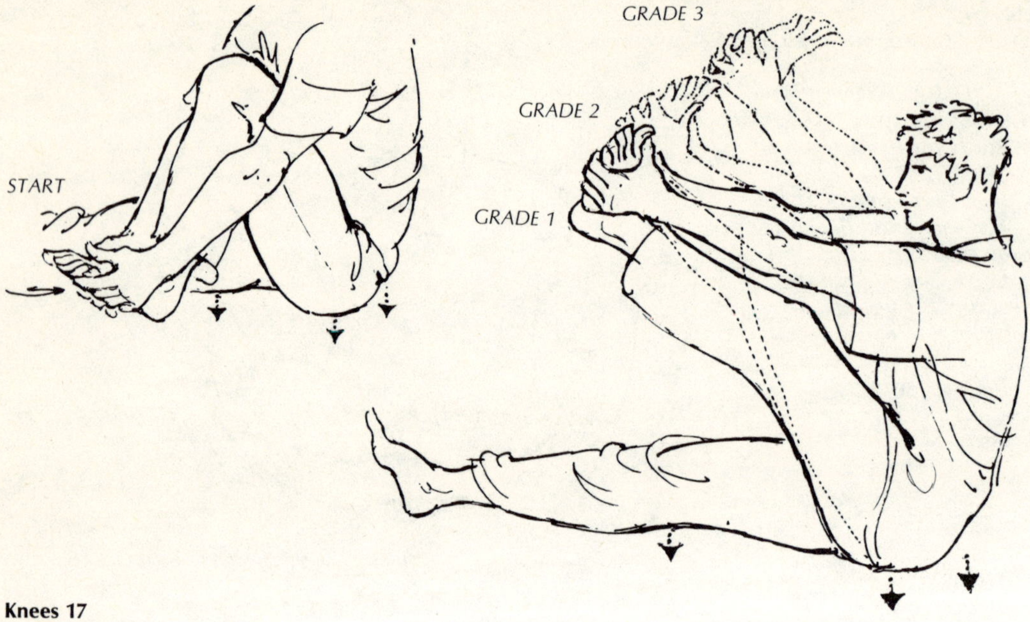

Knees 17

Start with one leg straight and one knee bent up with both hands holding the foot of your bent leg.

Exhale a few times down into your pelvis and slowly lift and straighten your bent leg.

Release and soften the skin at the back of your bent knee each time you exhale.

Eventually the knee will straighten as in Grade 2 and move higher as in Grade 3.

N.B. The more you are able to sense heaviness in your pelvis and opposite leg, the freer and softer the raised leg will feel.

Practise and release for 6 breaths.

Knees 18

With your back supported on a large cushion, bend up one knee and hold your foot.

Make sure all of your pelvis and lower back are on the floor.

As you exhale, feel very heavy in your pelvis and slowly start to straighten your leg.

Work softly and be content with a slight stretch behind the knee.

Try to release the sensation of tension consciously each time you exhale.

Eventually Grade 2 will become possible and after a while you can dispense with the cushion entirely.

Practise for at least 6 breaths.

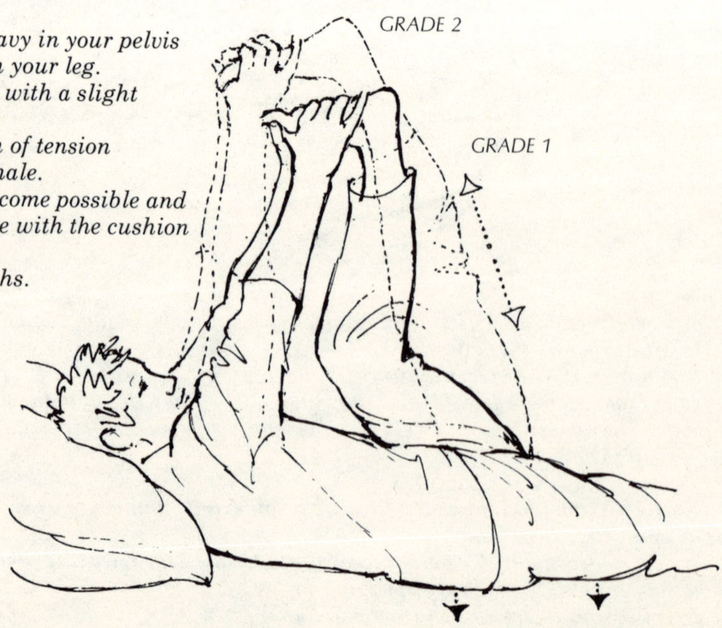

Knees 19

Pull one heel into your pubic bone and gently ease down towards the straight leg to stretch behind the knee.

Use a strap or belt if necessary.

Each time you exhale, feel heavy in the pelvis and equal weight through both buttocks.

Don't pull yourself forward, simply release and lengthen your spine towards the end of each exhalation.

Slowly, with practice, your trunk will close down towards your knee.

Practise for 8 breaths and then change sides.

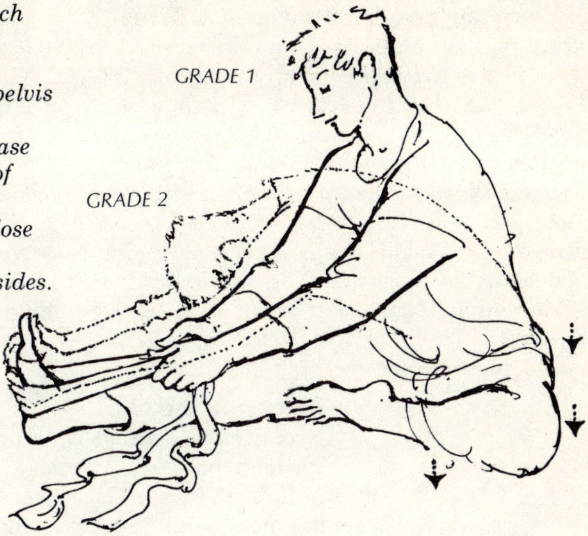

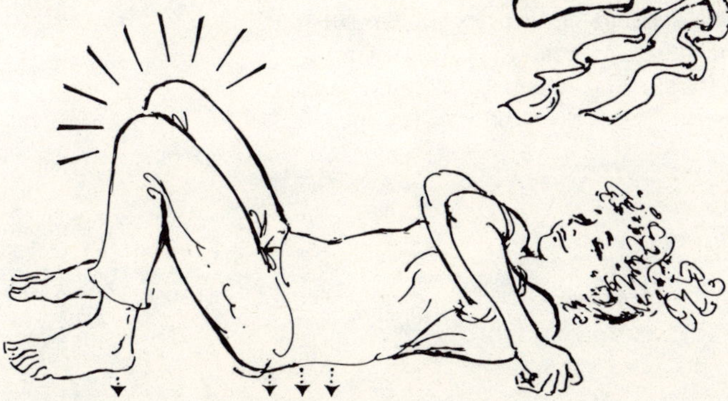

Knees 20

If you have worked specifically through a "knee" session, lie in the LRP and concentrate on the feeling in and around your knees.

Still allow your pelvis and lower back to sink during each exhalation. Try and sense your knees as softer, warmer, lighter and more clearly defined in your mind's eye.

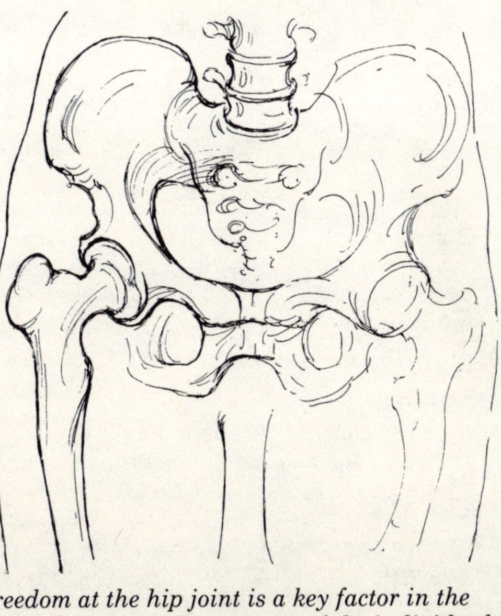

Freedom at the hip joint is a key factor in the free and integrated movement of the individual.

The Hips

In terms of freedom and balance the hips are probably the most important joints in the body. This is due to their central position, their relation to the pelvis and their great natural mobility and versatility of movement. The strong and simple ball and socket joint of the hip is designed for movement in all directions and its surfaces fit so perfectly that small defects easily influence general posture and even when sitting can throw strain upon other joints. Even though they function as a pair, the hips are rarely symmetrical. Differences may exist at birth, but more often result from postural maladjustment. Many people, when lying on their backs with their legs straight, have one foot turned out more to one side than the other, indicating that rotation is greater in one hip. Most people habitually cross their legs in one direction, indicating that one hip is freer than the other. And many habitually stand with weight resting over one hip which leads to and is a result of asymmetry. Because the hip structure is so stable, it is rarely injured in sporting accidents or daily traumas. But it is such an important weight-bearing joint that its integrity has a marked effect on its own long-term fitness and the fitness of less stable areas such as the pelvic and lower back joints. The hip undergoes hard wear and tear and is particularly prone to arthritis in later life. It loses its shock-absorbing power when its muscles are tight and out of balance and the lack of resilience causes the shock of leg movements to be exaggerated through the spine.

Three joints determine movement in the leg: the hip, the knee and the ankle. With so many moving surfaces there is potential for a great variety of maladjustments. Trouble below inevitably causes problems in the hip itself. The hips in turn co-ordinate with the pelvis and pelvic freedom at the hip joints is a key factor in the free and integrated movement of the individual.

Releasing the Hips

Because of the great versatility and natural freedom of the hips, there are many techniques that can be used to release and balance them. They are all worth trying.

Hips 1

From the SRP imagine your pelvis as a concertina with pleats at the front and pleats at the back.

Each time you exhale, imagine the pleats at the front closing and those at the back opening.

After a little practice you can feel your thighs rotating slightly inward at the hip joints.

Then reverse the imagery, sense the pleats opening at the front and closing at the back.

With practice you can sense the thighs rotating slightly outward at the hip joint.

This technique will make you even more aware of the fact that structure responds to "subtlety" and give you an inner sense of your hips.

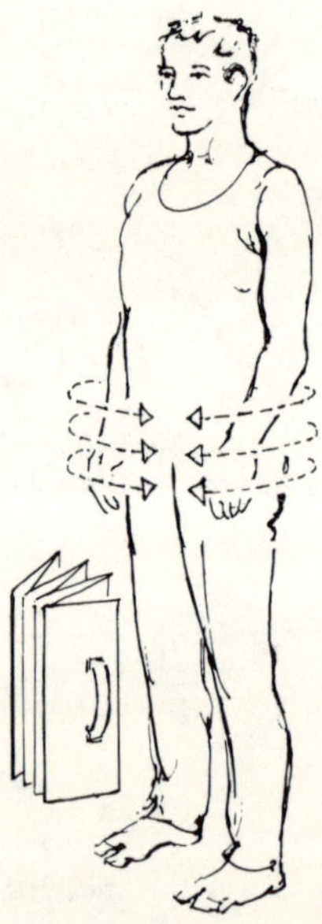

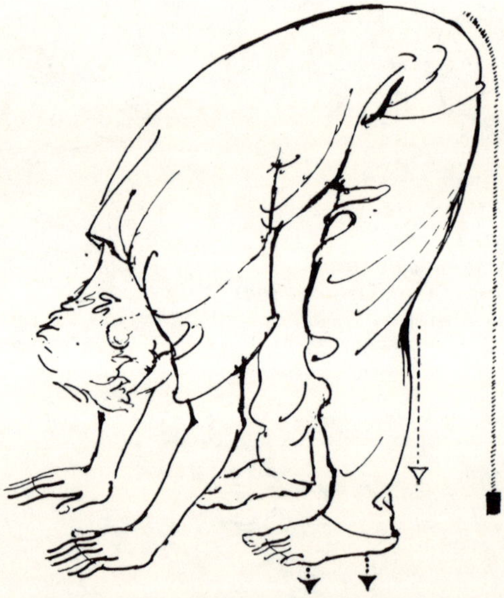

Hips 2

Simply bend your knees slightly and hang from the previous position. Each time you exhale, imagine the back of your pelvis broadening and your spine lengthening.

Release and relax your spine towards the end of each exhalation.

Release, lengthen and broaden for 6 to 8 breaths and come up slowly, exhaling through the heels.

N.B. *Take strain off the back by visualising a rope attached to your tail bone being pulled downwards to an imaginary spot between your heels, during the technique and when coming up.*

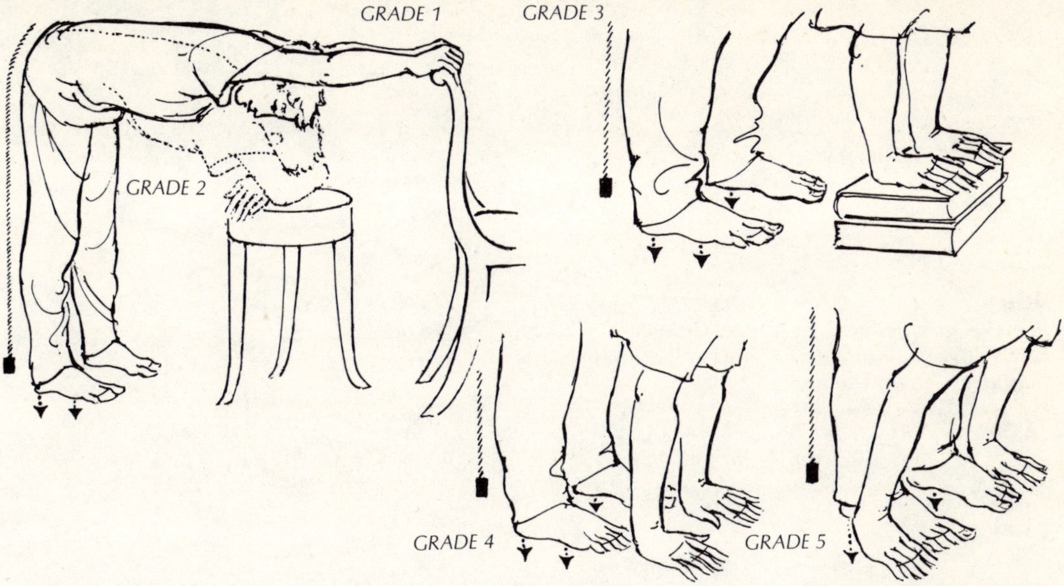

Hips 3

This well-known forward bending technique can be used for releasing the hips as well as the knees and spine.

Releasing the hamstring muscles at the back of the thigh is essential for structural freedom at the hip.

The grading is obvious—Grade 1 for those with tight hamstrings, through to 4 and 5 for the more flexible.

In all grades start bending from the SRP and each time you exhale imagine:

- *the tailbone being pulled down towards the imaginary spot between your heels*
- *the back of the knees softening and widening*
- *and your pelvis broadening across the back.*

Release the spine and shoulders towards the end of each exhalation to increase the movement at your hip joints.

Hips 4

From the SRP turn your right foot directly outwards to the right and the left foot halfway in the same direction.

Imagine your tail bone being pulled down to your left heel and keep most of your weight through your left foot.

Bend your trunk to the right as you exhale.

Keep your weight through your left leg and each time you exhale concentrate on:

- *the downward pull of the tail bone*
- *the left foot feeling very large and being sucked into the floor*
- *releasing your right shoulder and lengthening your spine outward and down towards your right foot.*
- *keeping the upper shoulder back to open your chest.*

Practise for 6 breaths and come up, exhaling down through your left foot.

Repeat on other side.

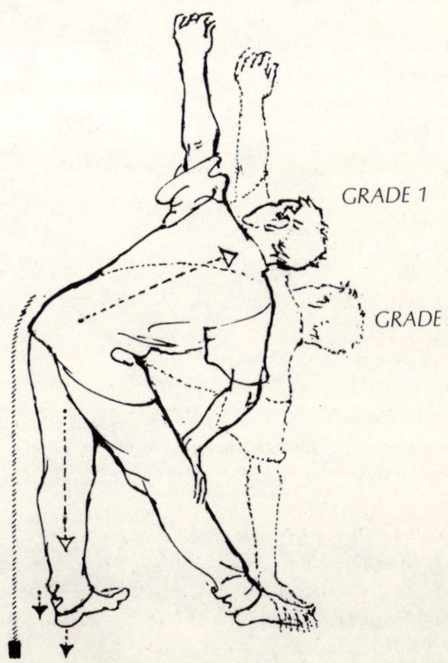

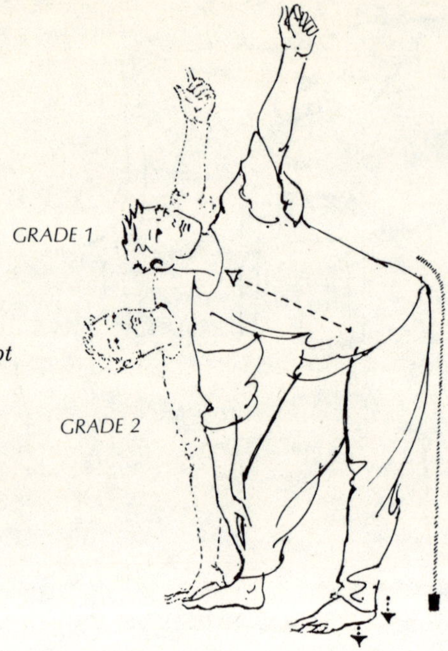

Hips 5

This technique involves exactly the same procedure as Hips 4, but the front leg is kept slightly bent throughout.

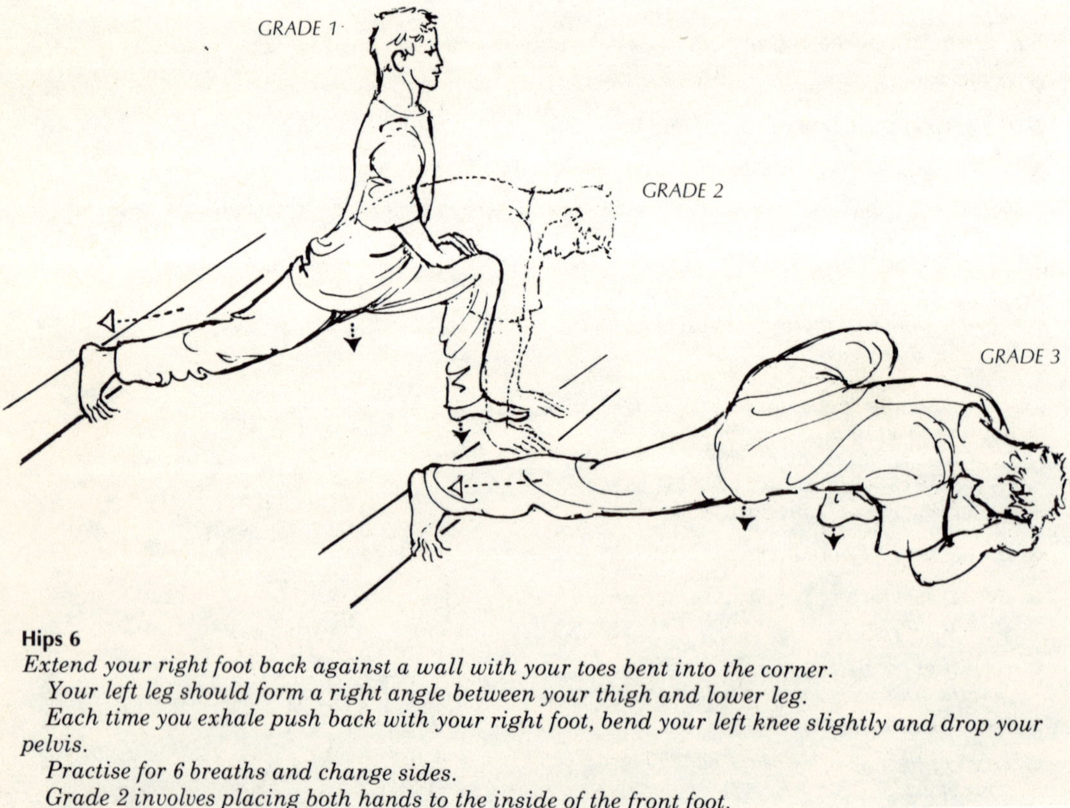

Hips 6

Extend your right foot back against a wall with your toes bent into the corner.

Your left leg should form a right angle between your thigh and lower leg.

Each time you exhale push back with your right foot, bend your left knee slightly and drop your pelvis.

Practise for 6 breaths and change sides.

Grade 2 involves placing both hands to the inside of the front foot.

Grade 3 involves placing both elbows on the floor. In this last grade stiffness in the hip may prevent you from placing the inner elbow on to the floor with ease.

Drop it softly as you exhale.

Hips 7

Place one foot on a table, ledge or desk.

The soles of your feet should rest comfortably on the table and the floor.

Exhale down through your lower leg and visualise your tailbone dropping and your pubic bone lifting.

Clasping your knee, slowly move your chest towards your upper thigh.

Practise for 6 breaths and change sides.

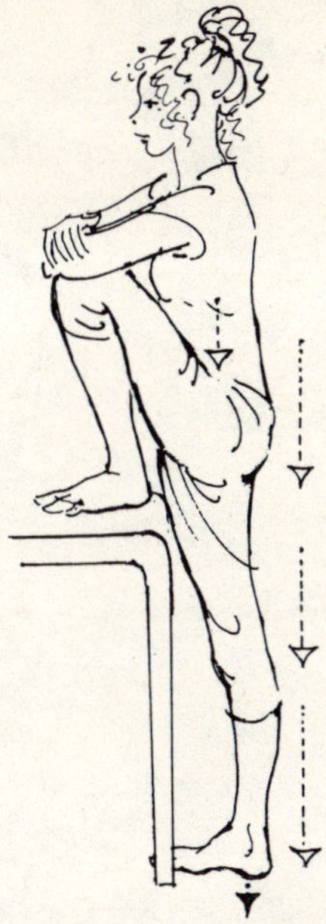

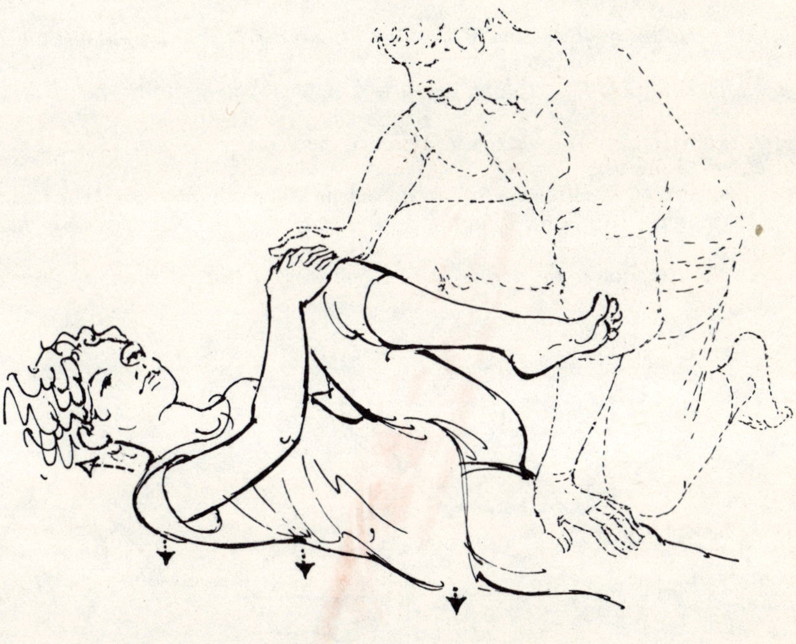

Hips 8

Lying down, pull one knee inwards to your belly.

Feel very heavy in the pelvis and the straight leg.

Lengthen the back of your neck.

Towards the end of each exhalation, hug the knee a little closer.

Don't force. Allow the whole pelvis to release.

In this technique you can use a variety of nuances, involving changing angles and leg positions. Be inventive.

Hold for 8 breaths, then change sides.

Another person can help admirably in this technique.

Work together in terms of slightly changing angles.

The pressure should always be downwards and slightly back towards the hip.

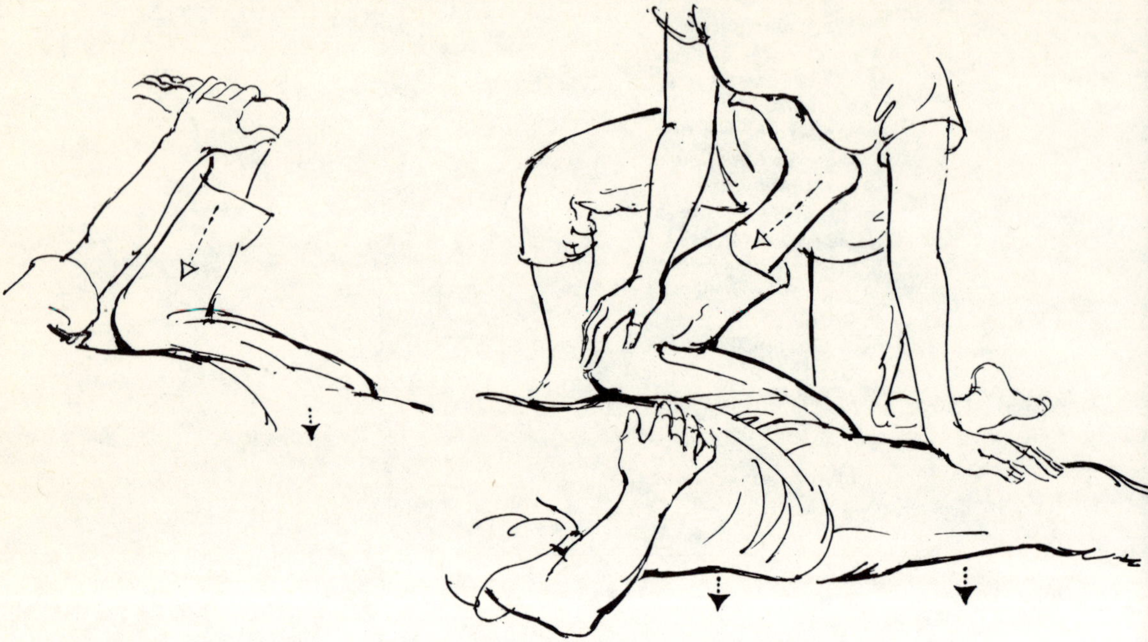

Hips 9
From the previous position, hold the inside of your foot and direct your knee down towards the floor at your side.

Try to keep the lower part of the working leg vertical and stay heavy in the pelvis and the straight leg.

Each time you exhale, move the knee a little closer to the floor.

Practise for at least 6 breaths.

Help from another person involves "getting in close" as shown in the second illustration.

The pelvis is fixed on the side of the straight leg and the foot of the bent leg can be nestled into the helper's armpit.

Movement is in the direction of the arrows. Grade the pressure for tolerance and release-ability.

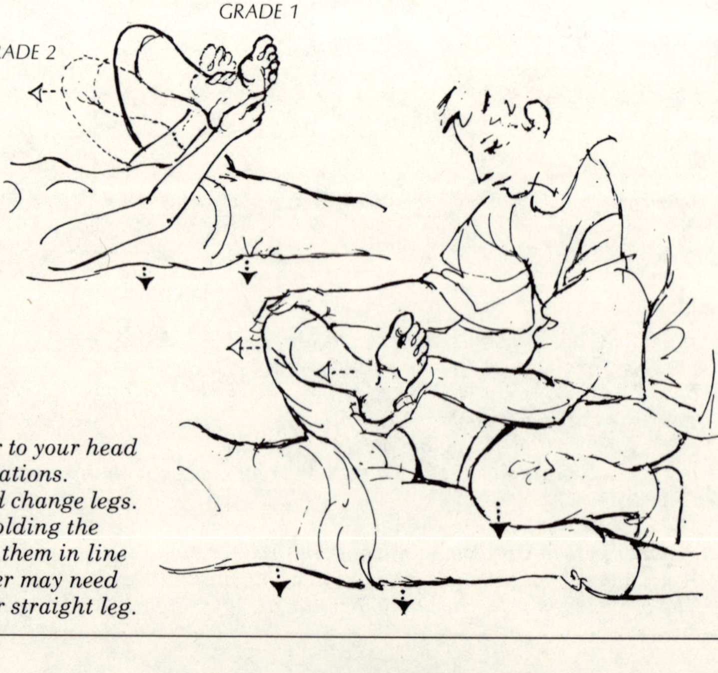

Hips 10
From the previous position slowly and gently ease your ankle and foot in the direction of your head.

Keep your heel raised about 15 cm above your belly and in line with your nose.

Keep releasing and feeling heavy in the pelvis as you exhale.

Only move the ankle closer to your head towards the end of the exhalations.

Work for 6 to 8 breaths and change legs.

A partner can be useful holding the ankle and knee and keeping them in line with each other. Your partner may need to use a knee to stabilise your straight leg.

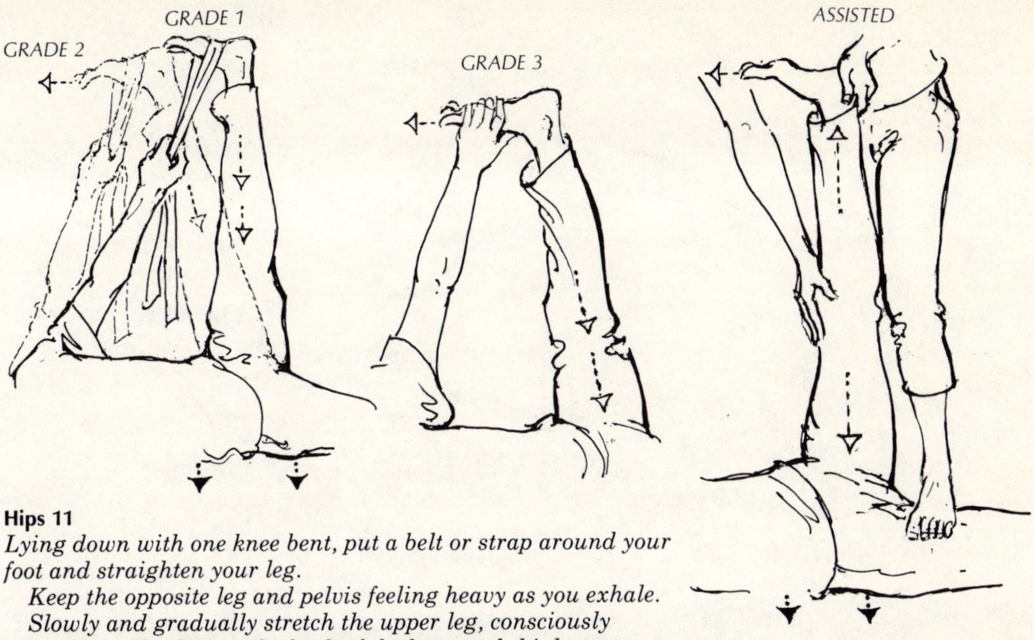

Hips 11

Lying down with one knee bent, put a belt or strap around your foot and straighten your leg.

Keep the opposite leg and pelvis feeling heavy as you exhale.

Slowly and gradually stretch the upper leg, consciously releasing and relaxing the back of the knee and thigh as you exhale. Grade 3 dispenses with the strap, though many people may not achieve this. Another person can be helpful in all grades.

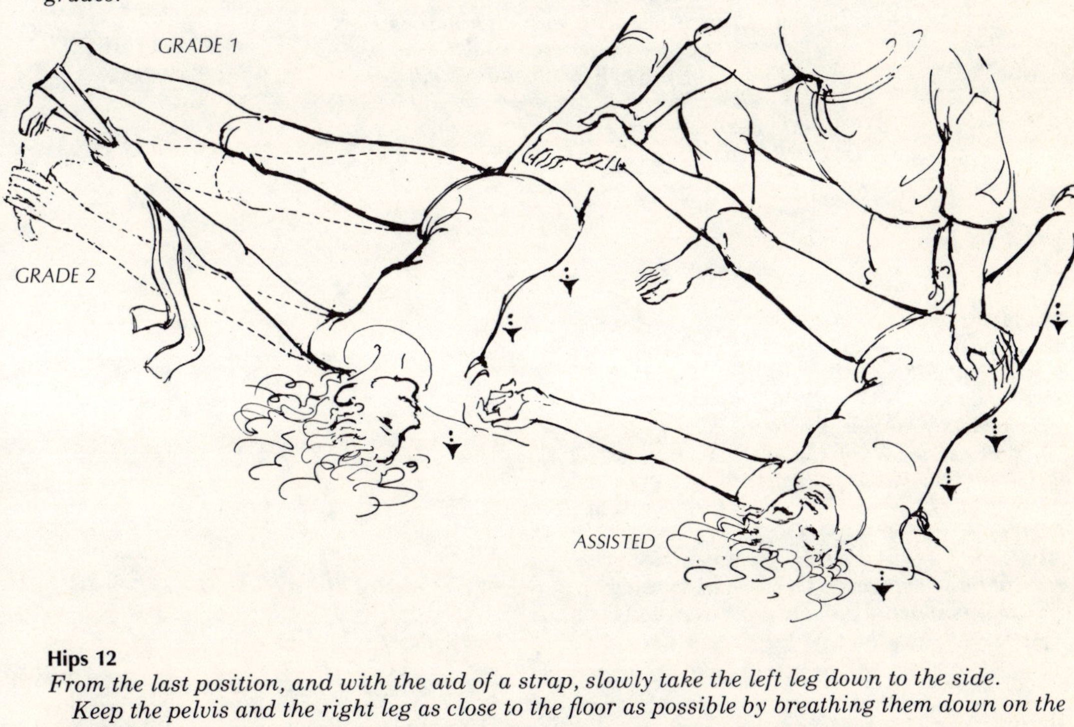

Hips 12

From the last position, and with the aid of a strap, slowly take the left leg down to the side.

Keep the pelvis and the right leg as close to the floor as possible by breathing them down on the exhalations.

Look towards your right hand and allow your left hip to release as much as possible towards the end of your exhalations.

Practise for at least 8 breaths.

Come up slowly and change legs.

A partner can assist by holding the opposite side of the pelvis in place and supporting the underneath of the outstretched ankle—it is more of a lowering than a pushing or a stretching.

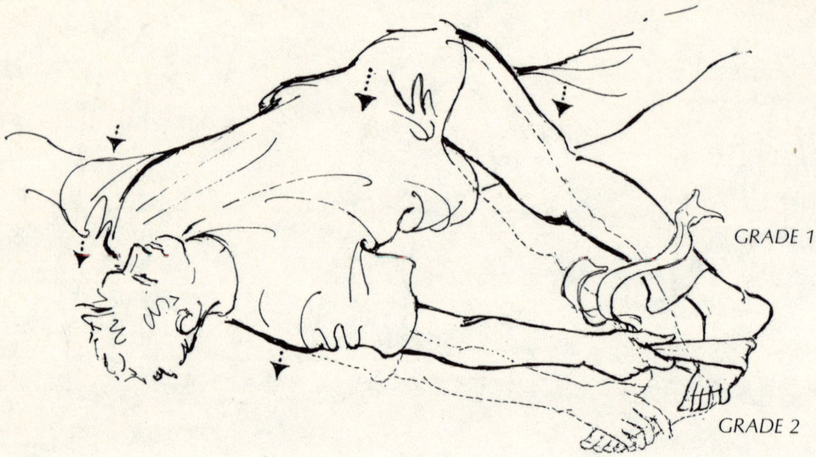

Hips 13
From the leg-raised position in Hips 11 slowly cross the leg over to the opposite side of your body.

If you are crossing your left leg over, hold your strap or foot with your right hand and look towards your outstretched left arm.

Each time you exhale, visualise your pelvis, both shoulders and your head sinking heavily into the floor.

Practise for at least 8 breaths on each side.

Hips 14
A very basic wall technique for tight hamstrings. More flexible people will find it unnecessary.

Keep your bottom well into the corner.

If your pelvis lifts off the floor, move slightly back from the wall as in Grade 1.

Keep your knees straight, your toes pointing down towards you.

With each exhalation sense your pelvis sinking into the floor and tension at the back of your legs softening and spreading.

At least 10 breaths.

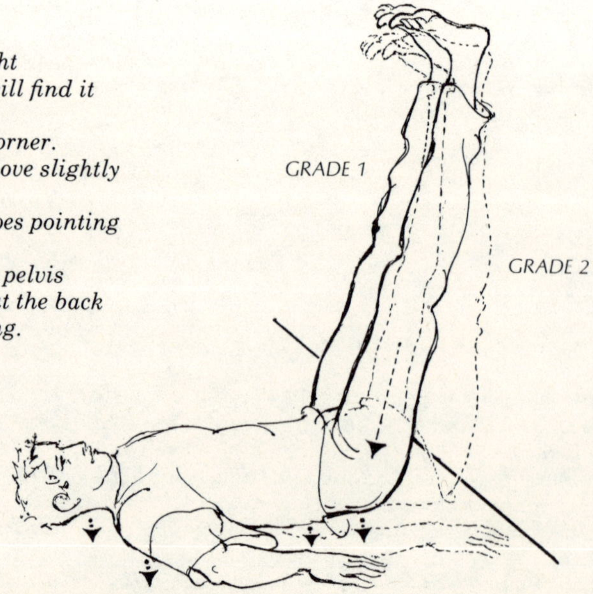

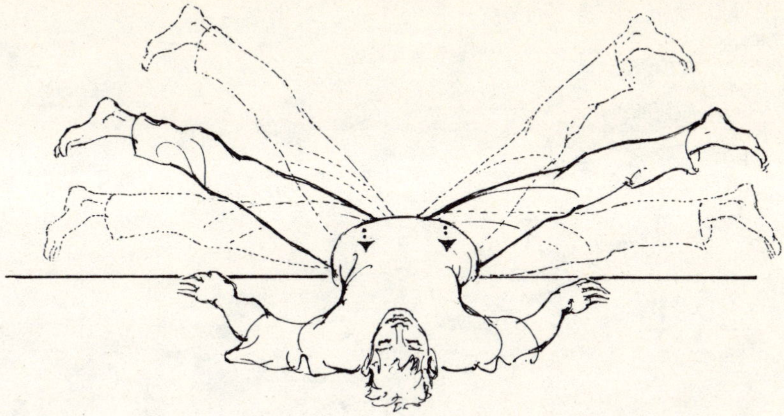

Hips 15

From the previous position, open your legs as wide as you can without forcing.

Keep your knees straight.

Allow the insides of your thighs to release slowly with each exhalation.

Concentrate on a sense of weight in your pelvis.

Sharp pain on the insides of your knees means you are overdoing it.

With regular practice you will be able to open your legs wider and wider.

It is worth holding this position for a few minutes.

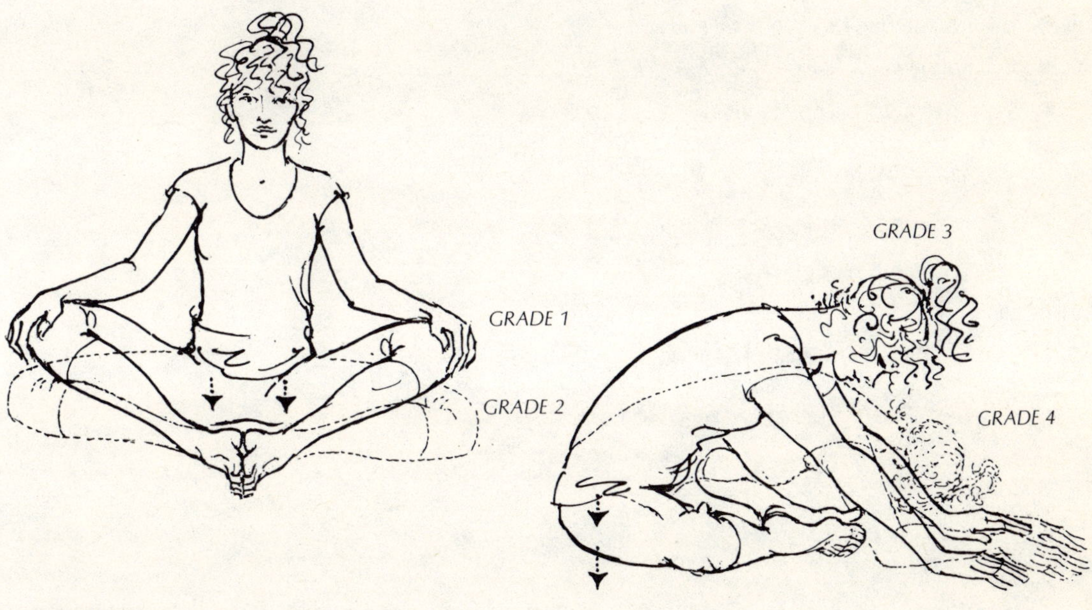

Hips 16

This traditional position is excellent for freeing and releasing the hips.

Sit in this well-known tailor position. If your hips and lower back are stiff use a wall for support. If Grade 2 is easy move on to Grade 3 and, when you are ready, Grade 4. Don't force in any of the grades and try to release consciously from the inside of your hips and pelvis each time you exhale.

Feel heavy in the pelvis in all grades.

If Grade 2 is easy you are already doing well.

As you move forward in Grades 3 and 4 draw in your belly towards your spine as you exhale.

At least 8 breaths.

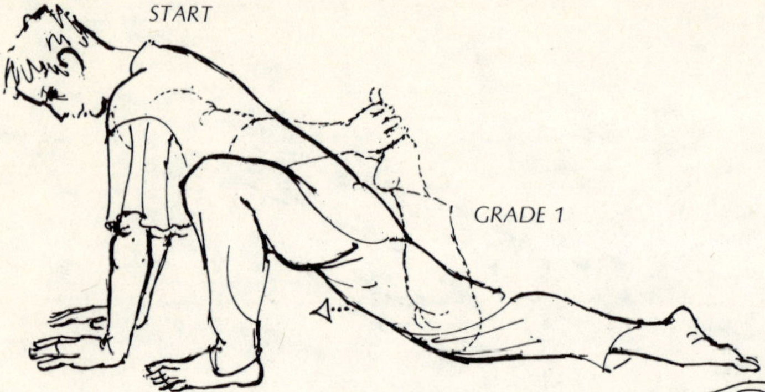

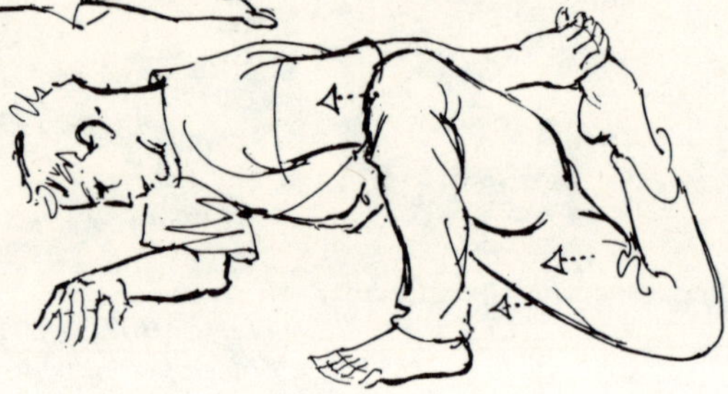

Hips 17

From the start position with the left leg forward, rest on your right hand and pull up your right foot with your left hand.

Project your front knee and your back thigh in the direction of the arrows.
This provides a strong stretch on the front of the back thigh.
Don't tolerate pain in the knee itself.
Consciously try to soften the area of most tension as you exhale.
The movement can be exaggerated by:

- *bending the front knee a little more.*
- *pulling the heel closer to your buttock.*
- *going down on your front elbow.*
  5 breaths are usually adequate.

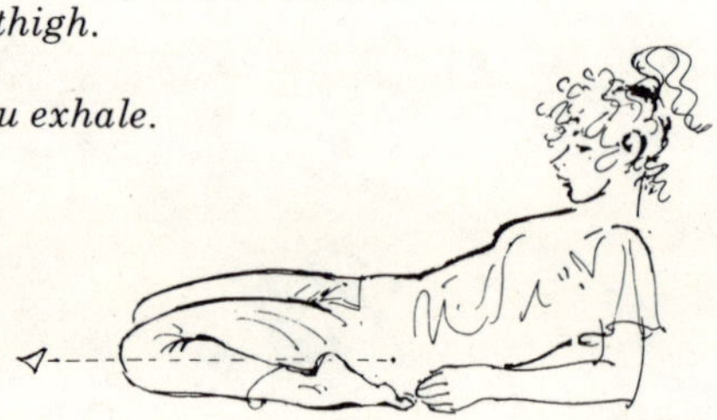

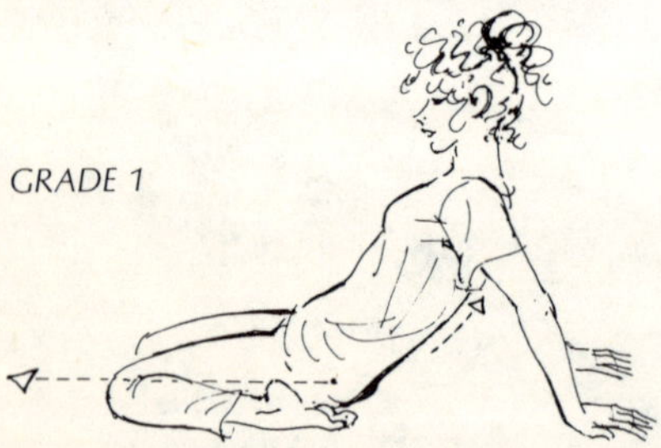

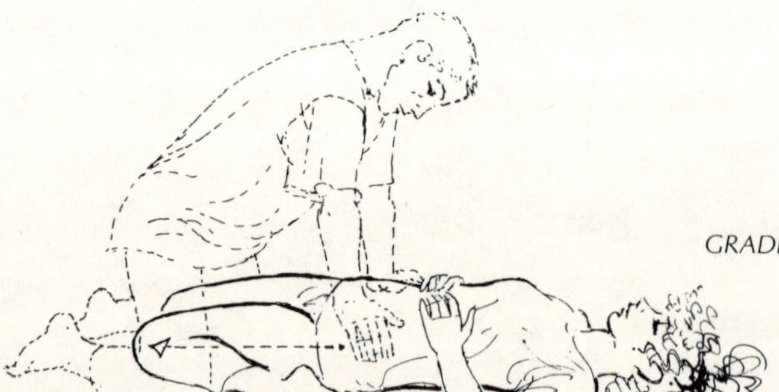

Hips 18

Again sitting between the feet, but this time to open the front of the hips. You have to work through stiffness in the knees and ankles first before your hips get the full benefit.

If your buttocks don't reach the floor in sitting, don't even try to lean back as in Grades 2 and 3.

Each time you exhale, imagine a line of movement from your tail bone to a spot between your knees.

Don't arch your back.

Keep your belly flat and draw it back against your spine as you exhale.

No more than 8 breaths to start with. Come up if you feel discomfort in the lower back.

Grades 2 and 3 can be assisted by fixing the pelvis and directing them as shown by the arrows, but they must always be released slowly.

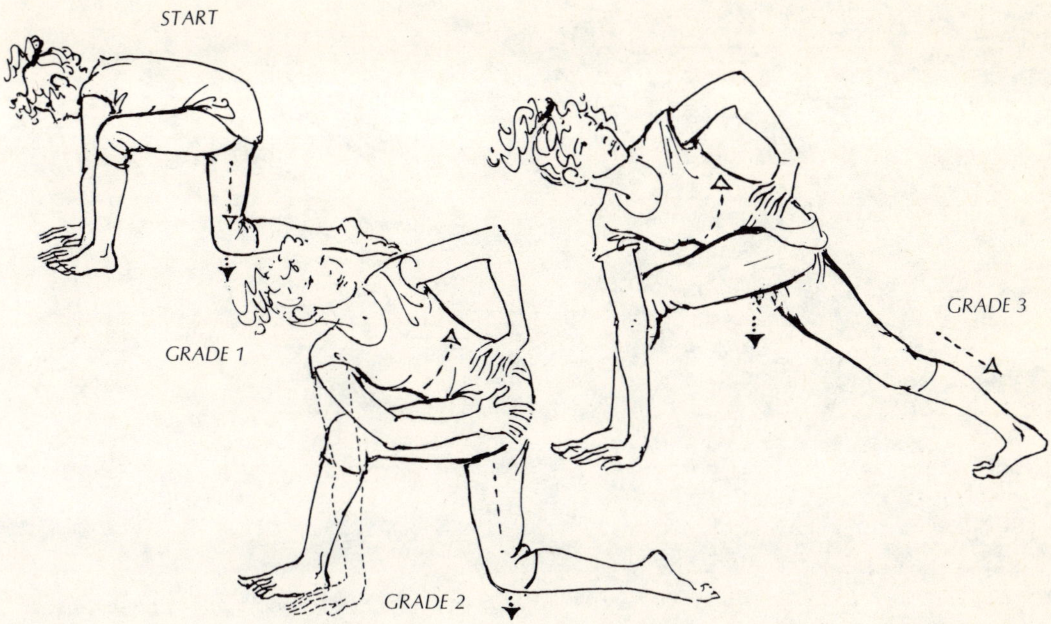

Hips 19

From the starting position with your left leg in front, feel heavy through your right knee and twist across your left knee using the back of your right arm as a lever.

Look behind you towards your back foot.

Release between your shoulder blades.

Exaggerate the twist towards the end of each exhalation.

Grade 2 involves sliding your right shoulder round a little more to place your right hand on the floor.

Grade 3 involves twisting a little further and raising your back knee—push back through your right heel for stability.

Practise for 4 to 6 breaths, then change sides.

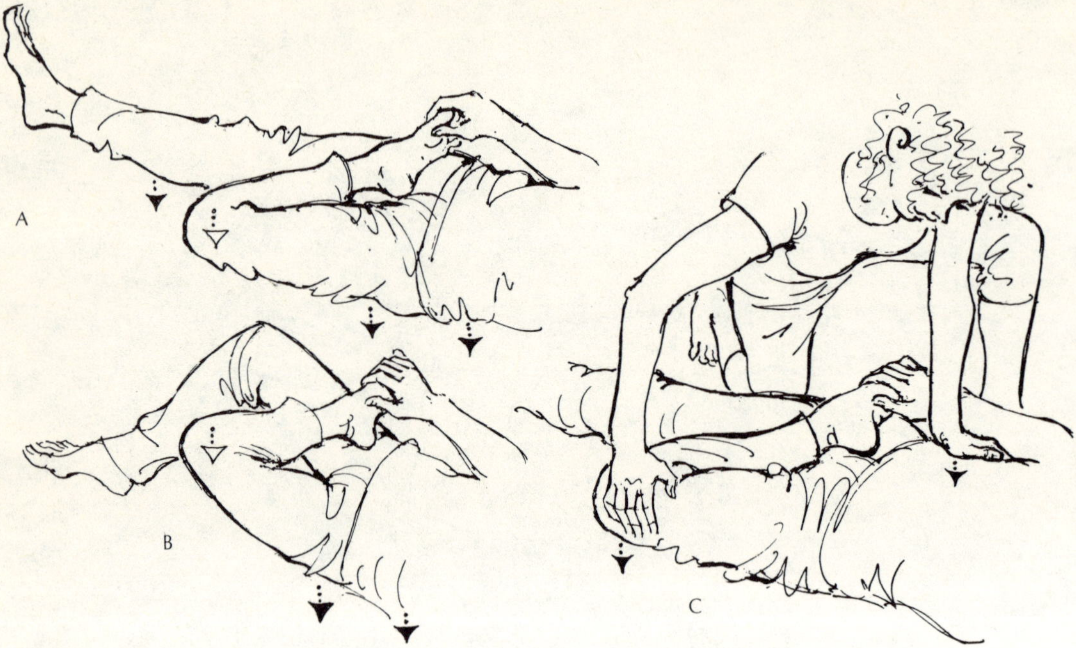

Hips 20

Lying on your back pull up your left heel so that it rests well up on to your right thigh as close to the upper groin as possible.

Hold the foot in place with your right hand.

Each time you exhale, allow the left knee to drop and sink slightly to the floor.

This opens the front and closes the back of the hip.

An alternative way is to bend up the straight leg as in B—this helps to keep the lower back flat on the floor.

Assistance from another person involves holding the right hip bone in place and guiding rather than pushing the left knee towards the floor.

6 to 8 breaths can be used in any of these three techniques.

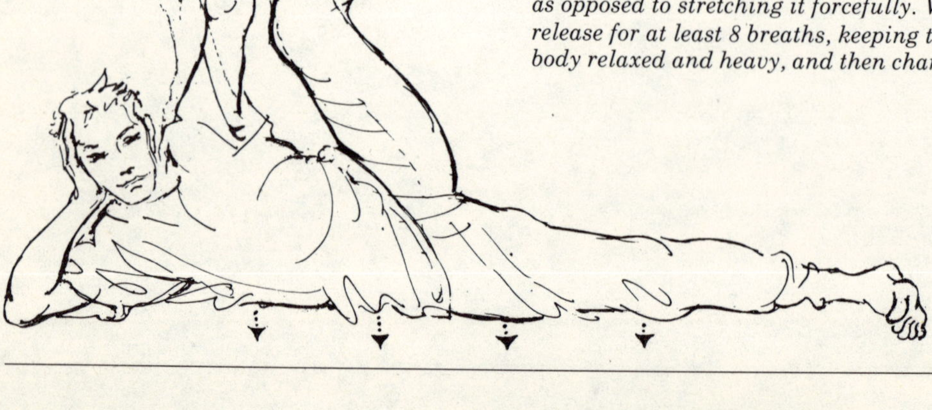

Hips 21

Lie on one side, head supported by your hand, and draw up the upper leg to hold your foot.

Exhale a few times and feel as if the pelvis is sinking into the floor.

Slowly straighten the leg towards the ceiling without forcing. Keep feeling heavy in the pelvis and releasing and softening the back of the knee each time you exhale.

Grade 2 involves straightening the leg completely but only by consciously releasing it as opposed to stretching it forcefully. Work and release for at least 8 breaths, keeping the whole body relaxed and heavy, and then change sides.

Hips 22

Sitting with the legs to one side like this is a good measure of, as well as a good technique for, hip flexibility.

It is important that the sole of the front foot contacts the inside thigh of the opposite leg and that the foot of the back leg turns out at the ankle.

It is surprising how few people can sit in this position with both buttocks resting evenly on the floor and sitting with the legs in one direction always seems to be easier than in the other direction.

Sit relaxed in this position for at least 10 breaths, allowing your pelvis to feel heavy and settle during each exhalation.

Repeat on other side.

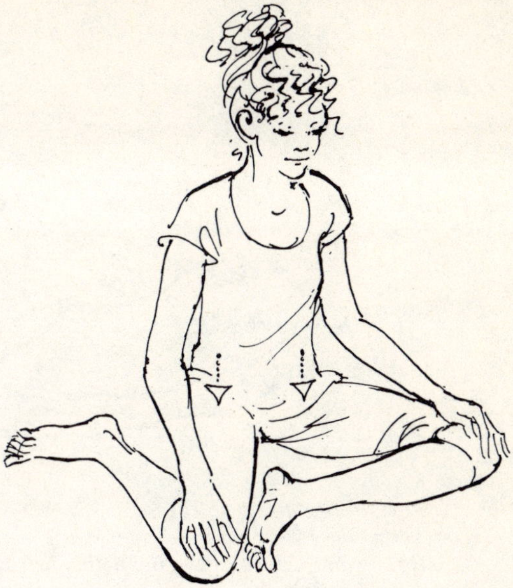

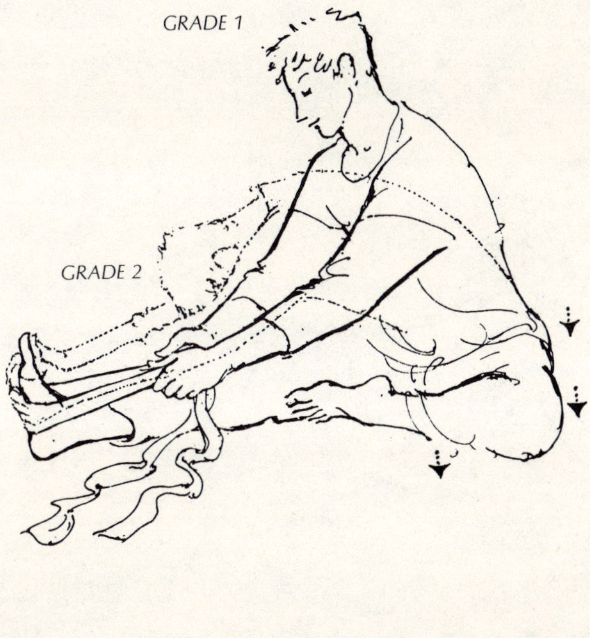

Hips 23

This illustration speaks for itself and the technique is the same as Knees 19 but with more emphasis on the hip joints.

It is important to feel very heavy in the pelvis as you exhale and to produce a sense of equal weight through each buttock.

Don't be impatient to get your trunk down too quickly—wait *for a sense of release in the straight leg before you extend.*

Each time you exhale feel broad across the back of your spine and the back of your pelvis and visualise a sense of deepening at the front of the pelvis.

It can also be useful to pull your belly back against your spine as you exhale.

At least 8 breaths and change sides.

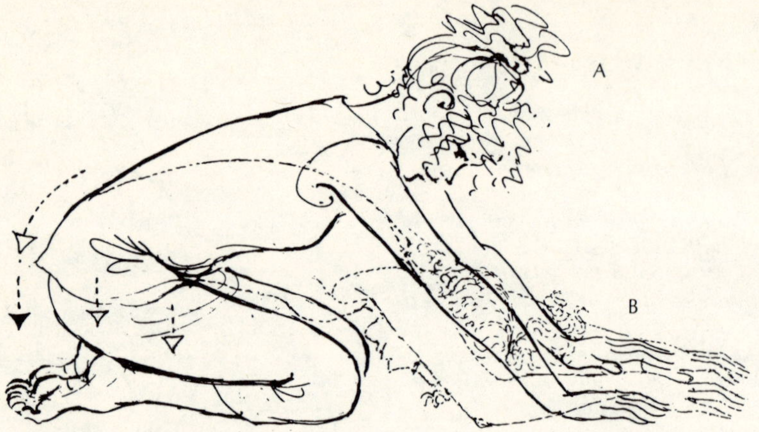

Hips 24

This simple fold-up position is particularly good for the hips.

Keep your knees together on or between your heels if this is comfortable.

Ease forward slowly, leaving the pelvis behind you as you do so.

Each time you exhale

- *release and relax the whole body.*
- *imagine your tail bone dropping down to the floor behind you.*
- *imagine your lower back opening.*
- *relax your shoulders and neck.*

Sink and release for at least 10 breaths.

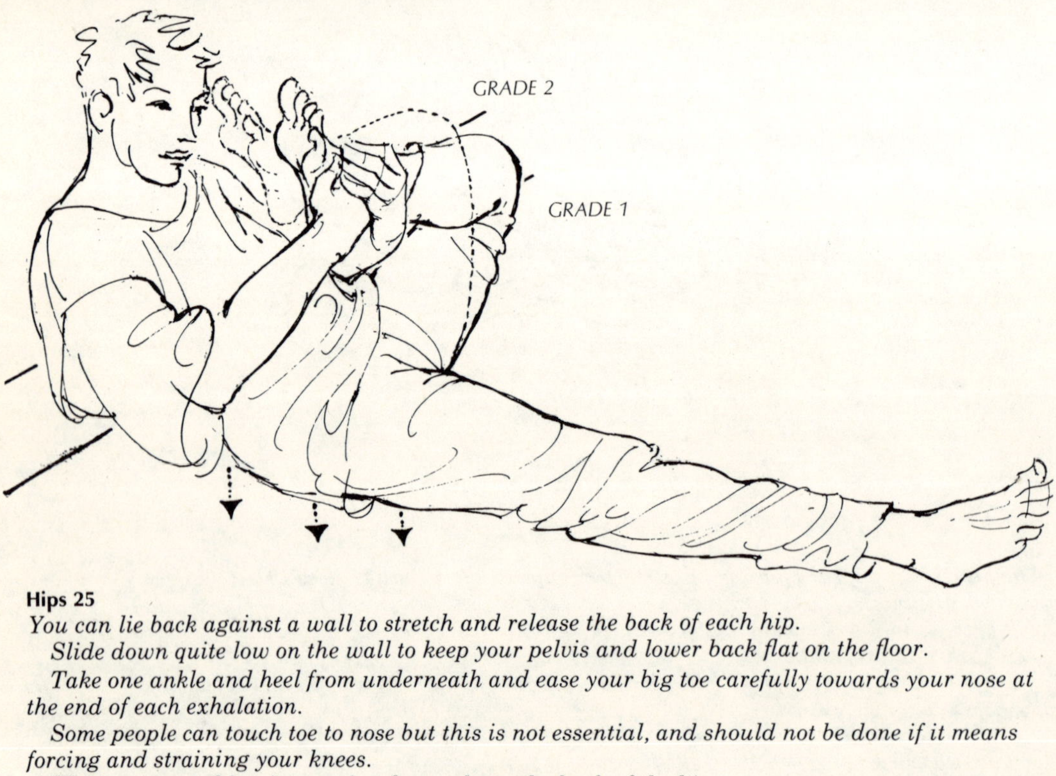

Hips 25

You can lie back against a wall to stretch and release the back of each hip.

Slide down quite low on the wall to keep your pelvis and lower back flat on the floor.

Take one ankle and heel from underneath and ease your big toe carefully towards your nose at the end of each exhalation.

Some people can touch toe to nose but this is not essential, and should not be done if it means forcing and straining your knees.

The important thing is consciously to release the back of the hip.

Work and release for at least 6 breaths on each side.

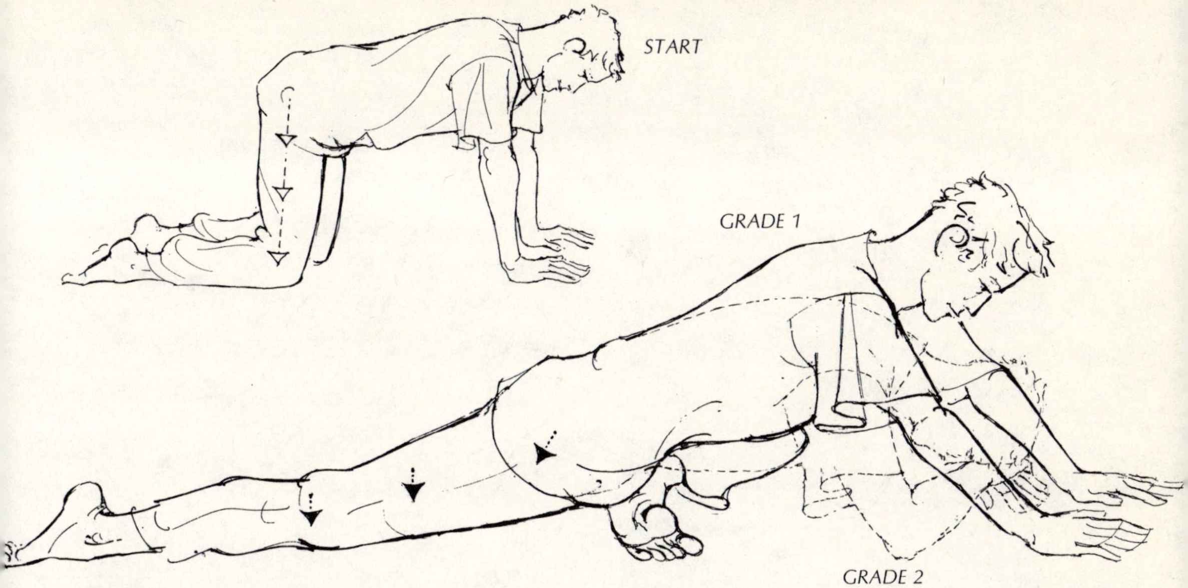

Hips 26

Again for the back of the hip.

From the start position stretch one leg as far as you can behind you, your front knee well out to the side to bring your pubic bone down behind your front heel.

Stretch your back leg far enough behind you to feel a stretch underneath the front leg or buttock.

Each time you exhale allow the pelvis to feel heavy and settle your whole body backwards and downwards behind your heel.

If Grade 2 is easy move your front foot further towards your chest. Release for at least 8 breaths on each side.

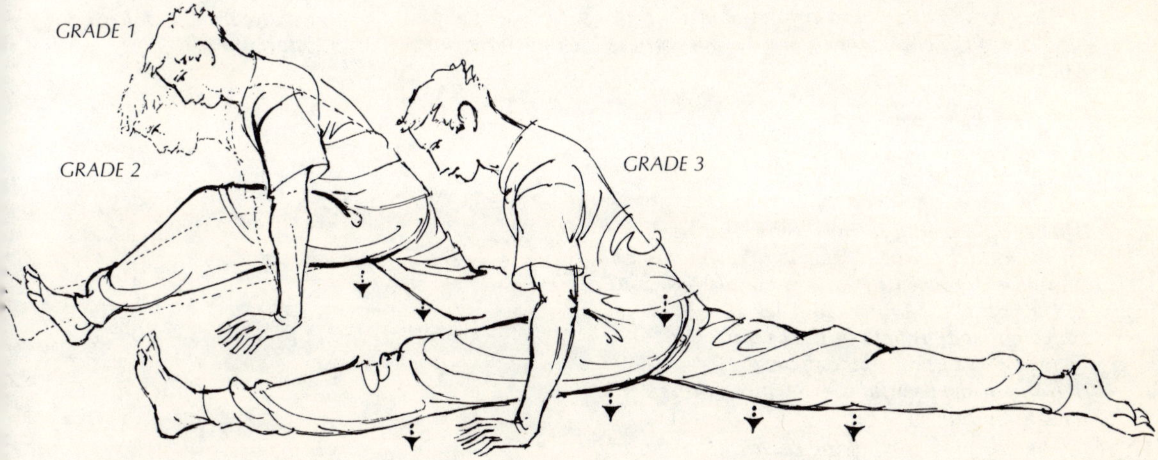

Hips 27

Try not to regard this as the splits (even though it is).

Even Grade 2 is advanced for people unused to structural work.

But the idea is to "release slowly"—extreme range of movement is not the immediate goal.

Simply support yourself well with your hands as in Grade 1 and eventually you will be able to lower yourself as far as Grade 2. This is not an essential technique, but is worth trying occasionally as all the other techniques will make this easier.

Practise this for as many breaths you can manage without straining.

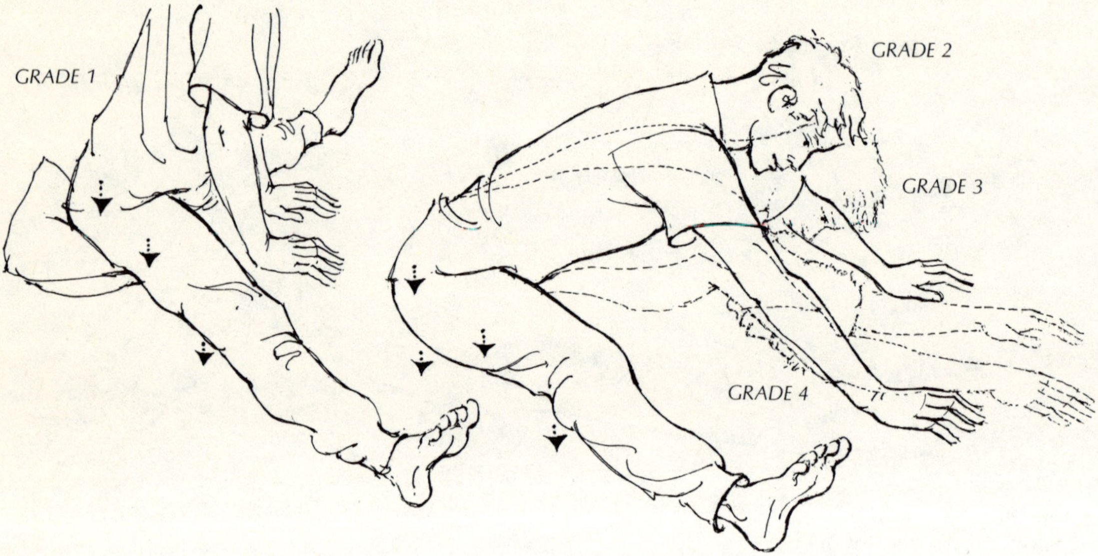

Hips 28

Most people should be content with Grades 2 and 3 in these side splits. It is a powerful technique and can provoke great resistance from the inner thigh muscles. Approached softly it can be most rewarding.

Spread the legs as wide as you can and if you cannot sit up straight, use a cushion as in Grade 1.

Each time you exhale feel very heavy in the pelvis and legs—and visualise the areas of most tension softening, spreading and becoming warmer.

Stay relaxed in the shoulders and neck.

Don't be impatient and try not to be discouraged as Grades 3 and 4 can take years to reach, and for some may never happen at all. The point is the quality *of movement, not forcing ranges of movement.*

Hips 29

This simple sitting release technique also used for the ankles again reflects how resistance and tightness are revealed by very simple positions.

The calf of the underneath leg should be well rolled out so that both buttocks have the opportunity to sink to the floor.

If this is too painful for the knee or ankle, put a cushion under the buttock of the upper leg.

The sole of the foot of the raised leg should be flat on the floor.

Gently hug your knee and take a few breaths to settle in this position.

Ideally you are working towards the equal pressure of both buttocks on the floor.

Even if this is easily achieved the position can be used with some slow exhalations to release the hip joints.

As many breaths as you feel suitable.

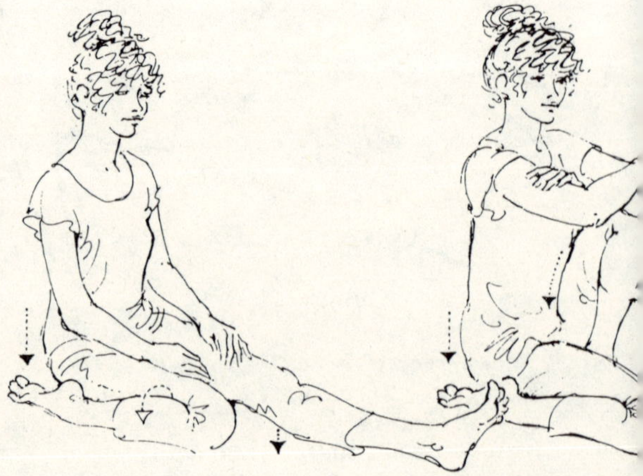

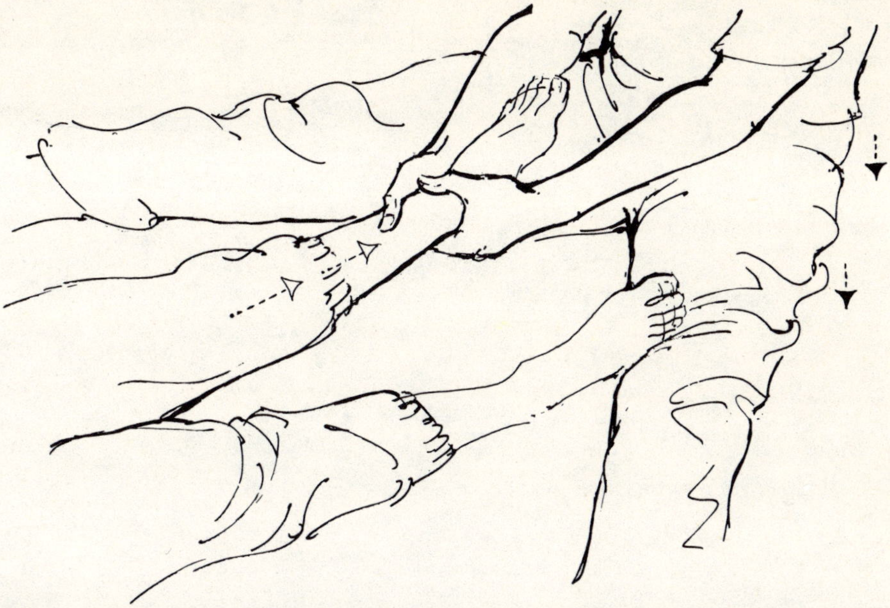

Hips 30

A partner can help to release your hips by simply pulling on your leg, clasping his or her hands around your ankle.

Your foot should be raised 15 cm from the floor and moved about 15 cm out from the mid-line.
Leaning back exerts a slow gradual traction through the long axis of your leg to your hip joint.
No sharp tugging or forceful movements.
The toes of your raised leg should point directly towards the ceiling.
Feel a sense of your hip releasing each time you exhale.
Try this technique for at least 6 breaths on each leg.
You can also try both legs together at some point.

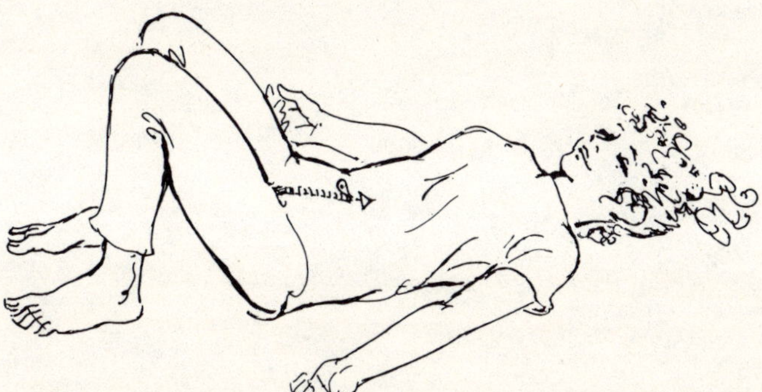

Hips 31

From the LRP but with your arms out to your sides and your eyes closed, imagine a zip that is hard to move being very slowly pulled up from your pubic bone to your navel.

At the same time visualise crinkles or wrinkles of imaginary jeans or trousers at the back of your pelvis being smoothed out.

Keep repeating the imagery each time you exhale.

This technique gives a sense of very subtle movement at the hips as the front of the pelvis closes and the back of the pelvis opens.

Use this imagery for at least 10 breaths and then relax.

The Middle Structure

The Pelvis

Balance and freedom of the pelvis is particularly important because its position and ability to adjust freely on the hips influences everything above it. Any unnatural tipping of the pelvis places a heavy strain on the entire spine. Some vertebrae may be crowded together and some wedged apart, some spinal joints may become compressed on one side and overstretched on the other. The very common exaggerated pelvic tilt causes strain at the junction between the back of the pelvis and the lowest lumbar vertebrae. This area is probably one of the most overstrained areas in the entire structure, as all forces tend to meet here. But when the muscles and joints of the hips and legs are in balance, this area is normally free from strain. Many therapists spend much time working away on the lower back and the back of the pelvis when they would do well to devote more attention to the hips. Some of the old schools of yoga worked solely on the ankles, knees and hips with the aim of freeing the spine so that a student could sit cross-legged on the ground without strain in order to practise breathing and meditation techniques. They were fully aware of the need for all the joints of the legs to be totally free before the middle and upper structures could find balance and harmony.

Positioning the Pelvis

All the techniques in this book directly or indirectly assist in freeing and realigning the pelvis in one way or another. However, these few simple techniques help to re-educate it specifically. The visualisation techniques can be "played with" almost any time and anywhere as they involve no voluntary movement. These techniques considerably reduce the angle between the lower back and the back of the pelvis. They should not be underestimated as few individuals are exempt from this common pelvic imbalance and this includes the unfit, the fit and the very fit.

Pelvis 1

From the SRP bend your knees and tuck your pelvis well under to bring your pubic bone as close to your navel as possible.

Feel your weight through your heels and the outside edge of your feet and keep your toes spread.

Slowly straighten your knees while keeping your pelvis tucked under.

Using 6 to 8 exhalations feel the back of your pelvis dragging downwards towards your heels.

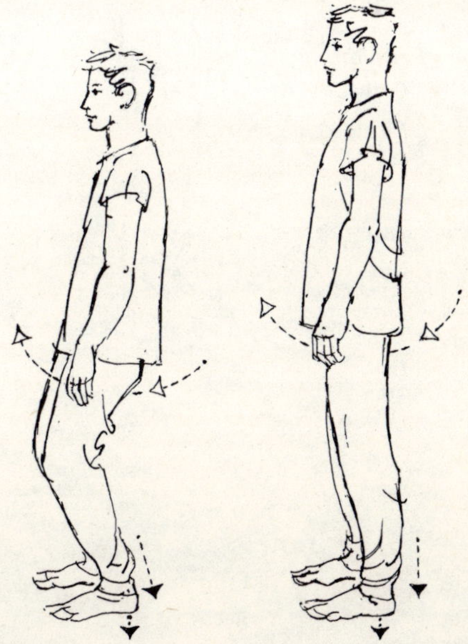

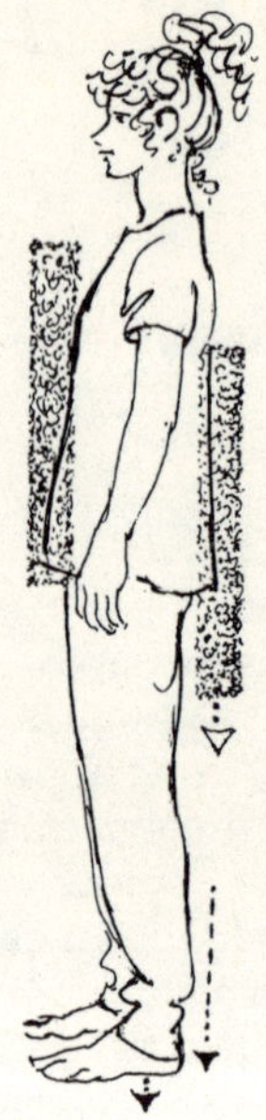

Pelvis 2

Taken seriously this visualisation technique can be very effective.

From the SRP imagine your trunk as a sandwich (heavy wholemeal bread). A large heavy slice front and back with a soft filling of your own choice in between, e.g. peanut butter, jam, tinned salmon or tuna, anything that in your mind's eye provides a consistency that doesn't quite hold the back slice in place.

Each time you exhale slowly, visualise the back slice slowly slipping down your back. The slipping sensation should start at the shoulder blades and end just beneath the buttocks.

Keep repeating the visualisation at the beginning of each slow exhalation.

With a little practice you can feel your pelvis tuck under on its own without any voluntary or muscular effort.

Visualise and release for at least 8 breaths.

Pelvis 3

From the SRP visualise a heavy, large-linked bicycle chain running down your back, between your legs, up the front of your body and over your head.

Each time you exhale, keeping your weight through your heels and the base of your big toes, visualise the chain slowly moving up at the front and down at the back in a continual circle of motion.

Keep the shoulders relaxed and released.

Practise for at least 8 breaths.

With very little practice one soon feels the pelvis lining up underneath the trunk.

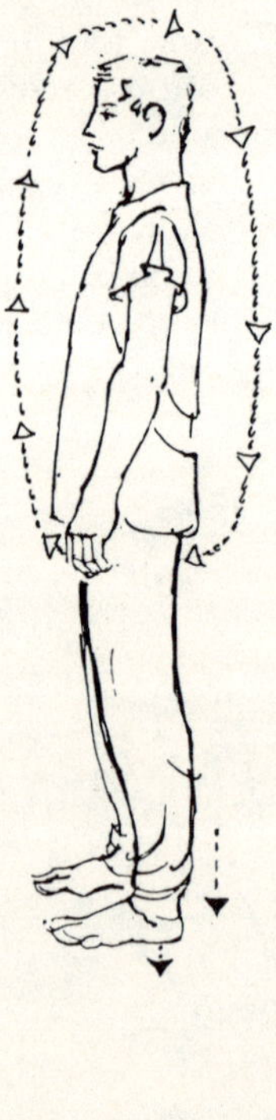

Pelvis 4

From the SRP and each time you exhale visualise a small person on the floor behind you pulling strongly and continually on a cord attached to your tail bone.

Visualise and release for at least 8 breaths.

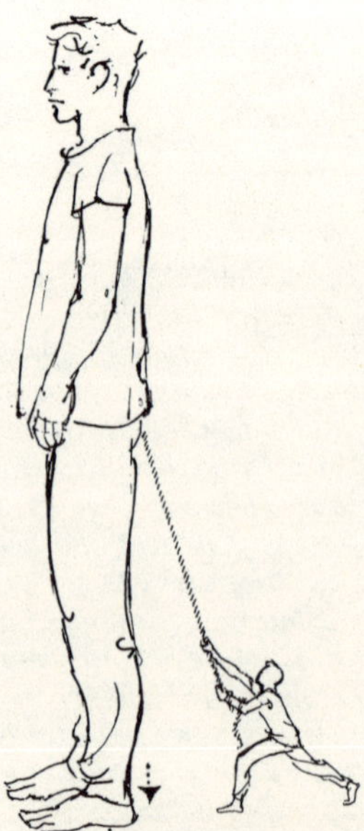

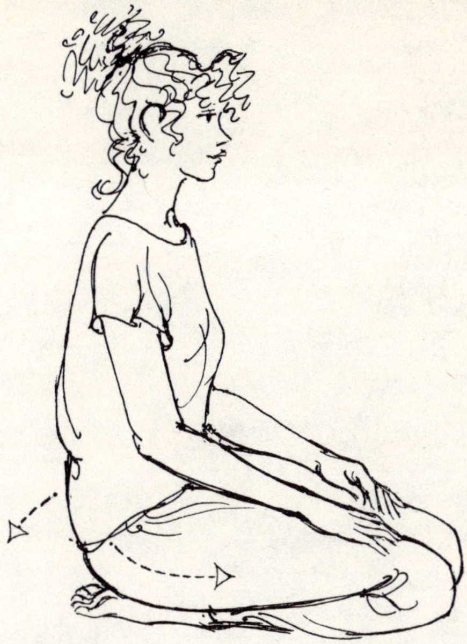

Pelvis 5
Simply sit on your heels and visualise your tail bone tucking under towards your knees and your lowest lumbar vertebrae projecting backwards each time you exhale.

Think broad across the back of your shoulder blades.

At least 8 breaths.

Pelvis 6
Stand in front of a mirror in the SRP and try and sense equal weight through each foot.

The weight should fall equally through each heel, the outer edge of each foot and the ball of each foot.

Look in the mirror and see if the pelvis has a tendency to shunt to one side, if so correct it and simply continue to stand exhaling down through the soles of your feet for at least 8 breaths.

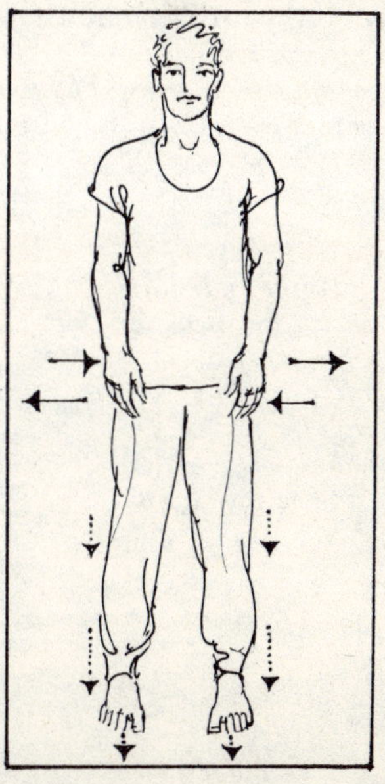

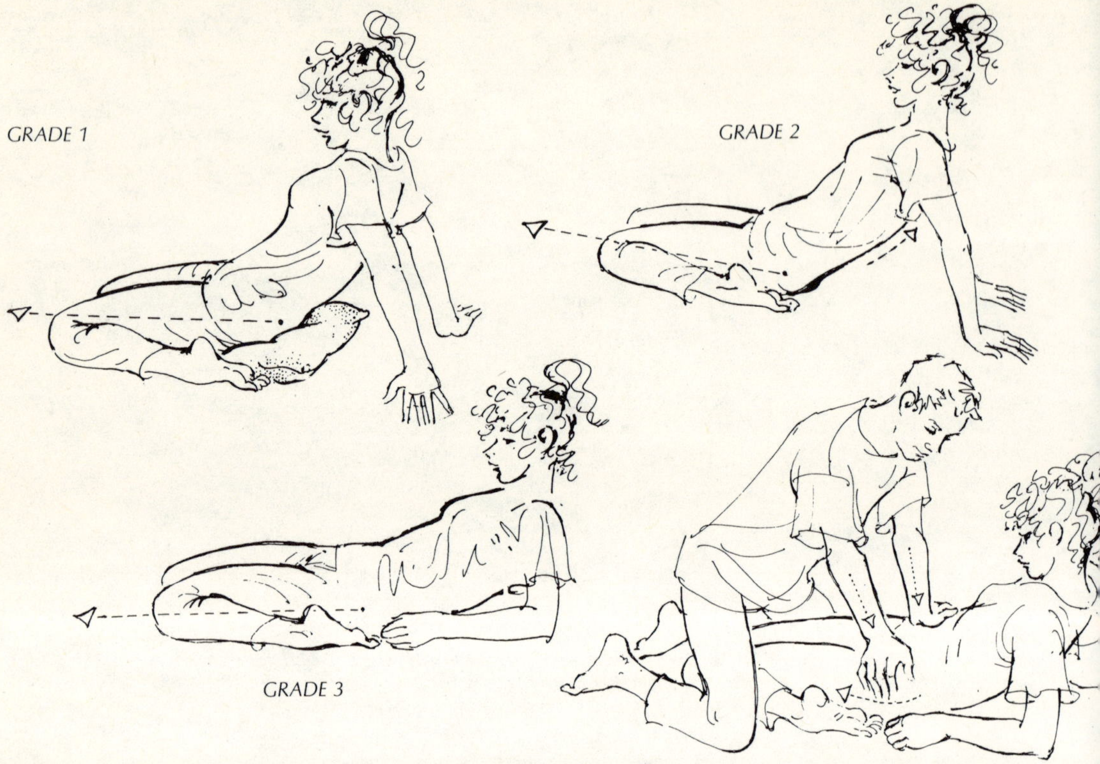

Pelvis 7

This technique, previously used in Hips 18, can also be used for positioning the pelvis.

Roll your calves out and sit between your feet on a cushion if necessary to avoid initial discomfort in the ankles or knees.

Imagine a line of movement from your tail bone to a spot between your knees and, keeping your belly as flat as possible, ease back on your hands.

If you need to use a cushion as in Grade 1, avoid going back on to your elbows as in Grade 3.

Avoid arching your back at all costs *and each time you exhale visualise your tail bone moving further and further towards your knees.*

Another person can be helpful by fixing your pelvic bones as you ease back.

The idea is that they assist in **reducing** *any possibility of the arch in your lower back.*

Pelvis 8

In the LRP imagine your tail bone being pulled towards your heels, your lower back and waist flattening and taking root into the floor each time you exhale.

Visualise and release for at least 8 breaths.

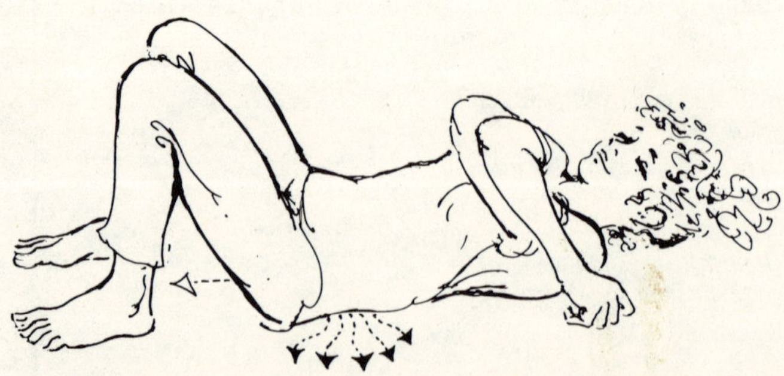

The Sacro-Iliac Joints

Most people who have visited an osteopath or chiropractor with lower back pain or sciatica will most probably have heard of these two joints at the back of the pelvis. But many people are oblivious to them, because their movement is hardly noticeable; you cannot move them at will or sense them in the usual way. The sacro-iliac joints are located between the sacrum at the base of the spine and the pelvic bones or ilium. The sacrum forms the back of the pelvis. The main function of the SI joints is to transfer weight from the spine and sacrum through the pelvis to the legs. There are various theories as to where the centre of SI movement comes from because the joints are a strange shape and it is difficult to analyse such small movements. The joints' surfaces vary from person to person and different types of movement occur in different people under different circumstances. In normal movement the sacrum pivots backwards and forwards between the pelvic bones and this changes the front to back measurements of the upper and lower part of the pelvis. For this reason the SI joints are important in the mechanics of labour and childbirth, and are more flexible in females, particularly during certain phases of the menstrual cycle and pregnancy. In elderly males they fuse together totally.

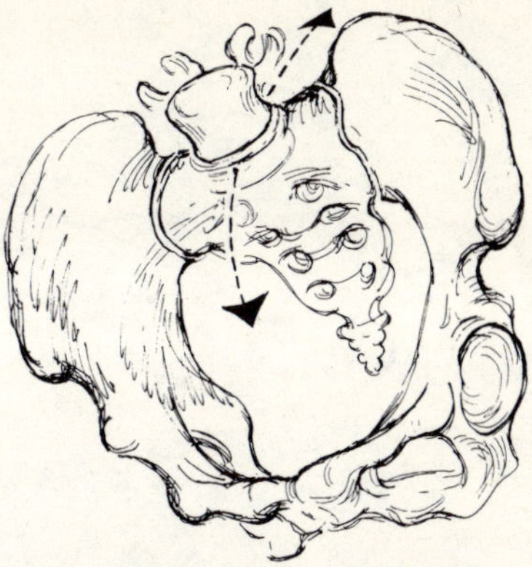

The sacrum pivots backwards and forwards between the pelvic bones.

SI balance is affected by pulls on the pelvic bones coming from the large thigh muscles below, the trunk and spinal muscles above, and pulls on the sacrum coming from the deep muscles at the back of the hip. SI strain is very common and the joints can be damaged in a variety of ways, sometimes producing very painful symptoms, and upsetting the balance of the spine above. The forward and backward movement of the sacrum is often disturbed and it can also "slip" into side bent and twisted positions. The SI joints act as a pair and when you stand and put weight on one leg, movement on one side is balanced by an opposite movement on the other. Habitually standing with weight on one leg or sitting with the legs crossed in the same direction causes a twist in the joints. Strain may also occur during extreme movements of the leg or trunk, when the muscles are tight and the SI joints are forced out of true. They are particularly prone to strain during pregnancy when the ligaments soften in preparation for childbirth. They are also prone to strain from imbalances and tightness in the legs, hips and lower back and when the natural spinal curves are exaggerated. However, when the entire structure is free and in balance the SI joints are less prone to injury and the sacrum itself is less prone to slipping or hitching.

Stabilising the Sacro-Iliac Joints

The following techniques are specific and seek to find a balance between opening and closing the sacro-iliac joints.

Sacro-Iliac 1

Start in the LRP and simply feel your pelvis broadening at the back, closing at the front and sinking into the floor each time you exhale.

Breathe slowly in and out through the nose and sink the pelvis for at least 6 breaths.

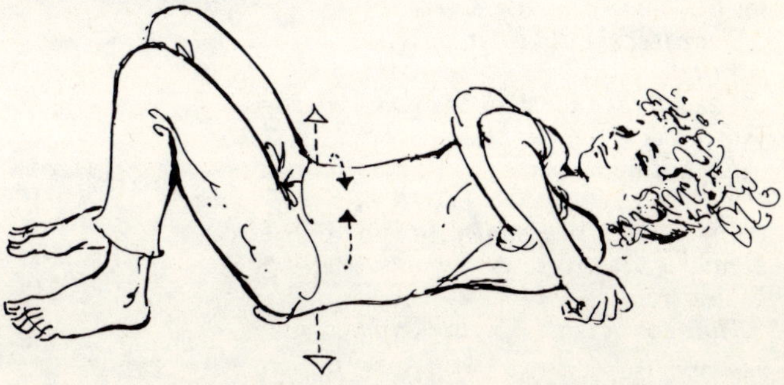

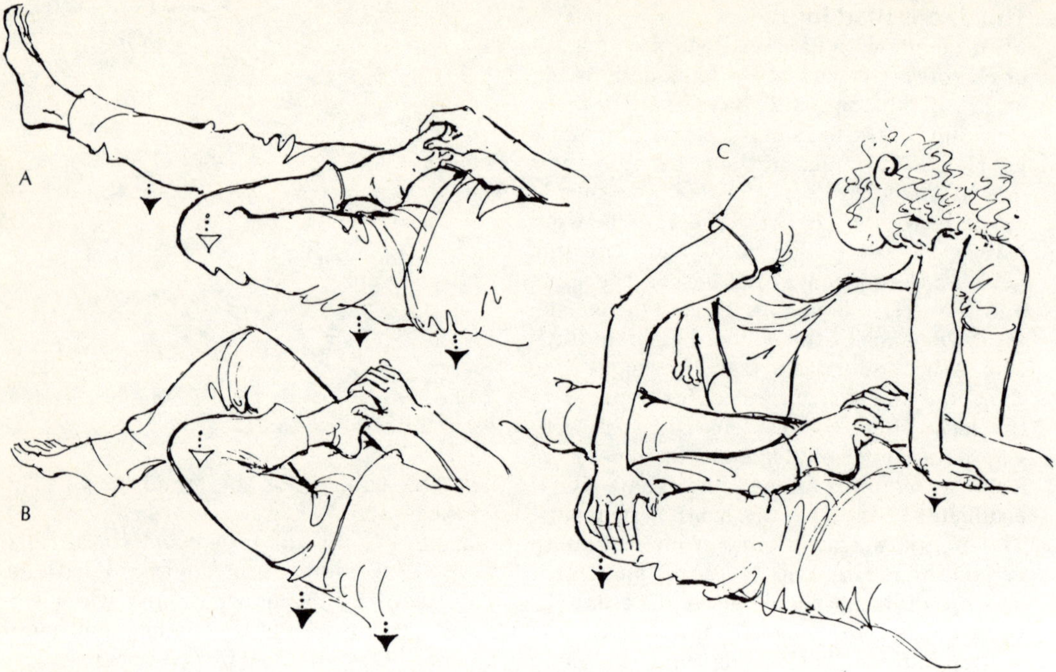

Sacro-Iliac 2

From the previous position, put one foot into position A.

This technique, used in Hips 20 to open the front of the hip, can be used for closing the sacro-iliac joints.

The instruction is the same except that you should focus your attention on the buttock of the bent leg closing up and reducing in size each time the knee drops closer to the floor during your exhalations.

Don't tolerate pain in your knee or ankle.

You can bend the opposite leg up as in B or use a partner to help you release as in C.

The person helping is not pushing but **guiding** *the bent knee down towards the floor while fixing the opposite hip bone.*

Try A, B or C for at least 6 breaths allowing the pelvis and both legs to feel as heavy as possible during your exhalations.

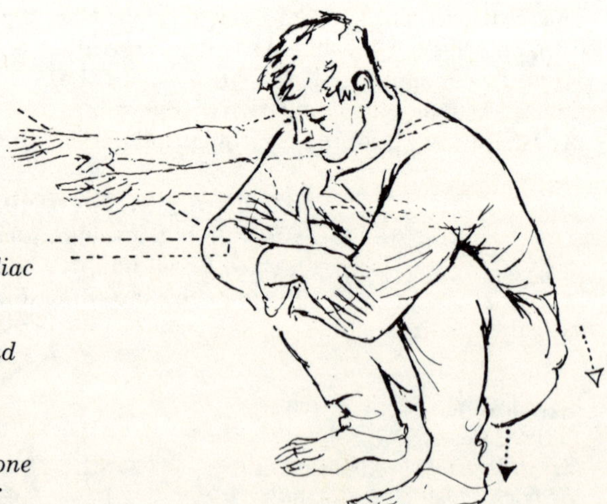

Sacro-Iliac 3

Graded squatting is also good for the sacro-iliac joints as it tends to drop the sacrum between the hip bones or pelvic bones.

Your feet should be at least 30 cm apart and parallel.

Use a folded towel or blanket underneath your heels if your ankles are stiff.

Each time you exhale, imagine your tail bone slowly dropping to the floor, the back of your pelvis gradually broadening and your lowest lumbar vertebrae projecting down and back behind you.

Hold for at least 6 breaths and come up slowly.

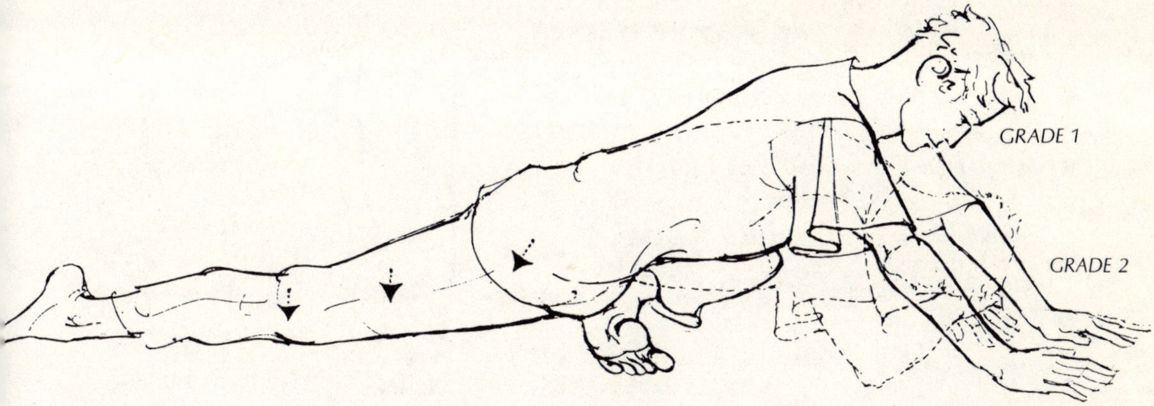

Sacro-Iliac 4

Hips 26 is ideal for opening and releasing the sacro-iliac joints. This is a particularly beneficial technique to remove residual stiffness resulting from a painful episode of sciatica. But be sure that the pain is gone before using the technique.

Follow the instruction in Hips 26 and release for at least 6 to 8 exhalations on each side.

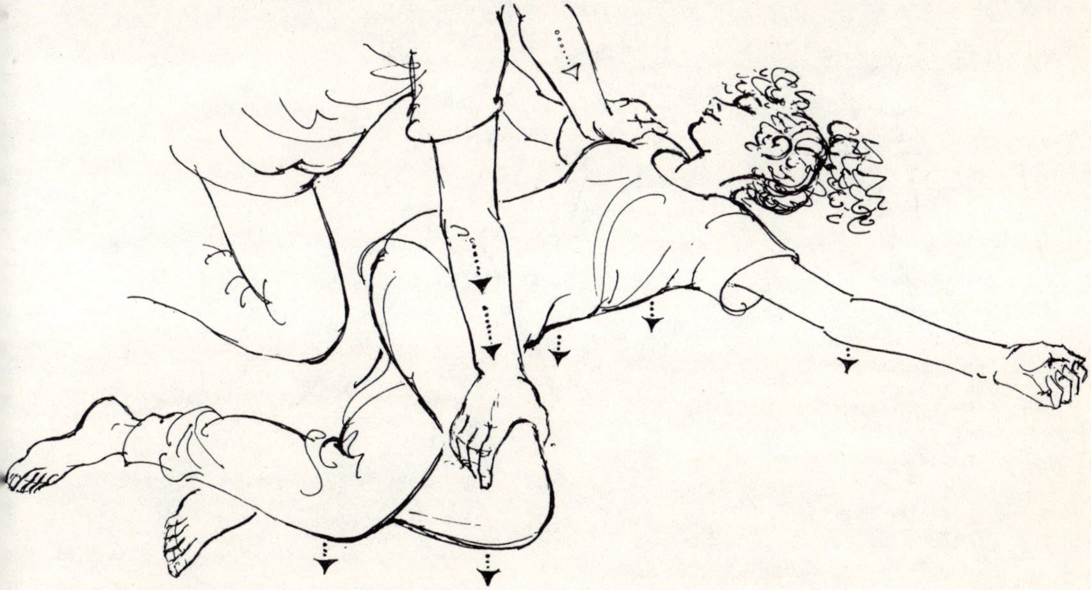

Sacro-Iliac 5

This popular floor twist needs to be performed with a very relaxed approach.

Keep both shoulders on the floor and your pelvis very heavy as you slowly take your upper knee down to its opposite side i.e. if your right leg is on top, slowly direct it down to the floor on your left.

Work slowly and release for at least 6 breaths on each side.

Any assistance from a partner should have a gentle and light touch and should involve the minimum pressure necessary to exaggerate the technique.

Sacro-Iliac 6

This common forward bend from the SRP is the same as Knees 2, but is only beneficial to the sacro-iliac joints if you have at least Grade 3 flexibility in that technique.

The focus is entirely on the back of the pelvis. Imagine:

- *the back of the pelvis broadening when you exhale*
- *the tail bone projecting downwards to an imaginary spot on the floor behind you.*

Remember to keep the chest and shoulders completely relaxed.

Work gently for at least 4 breaths and come up slowly.

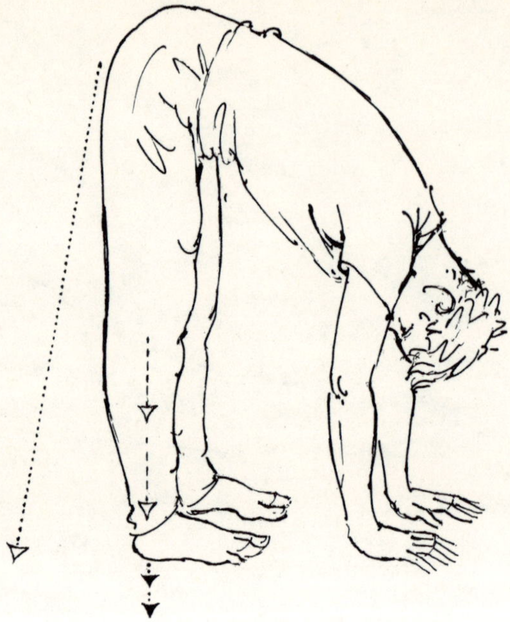

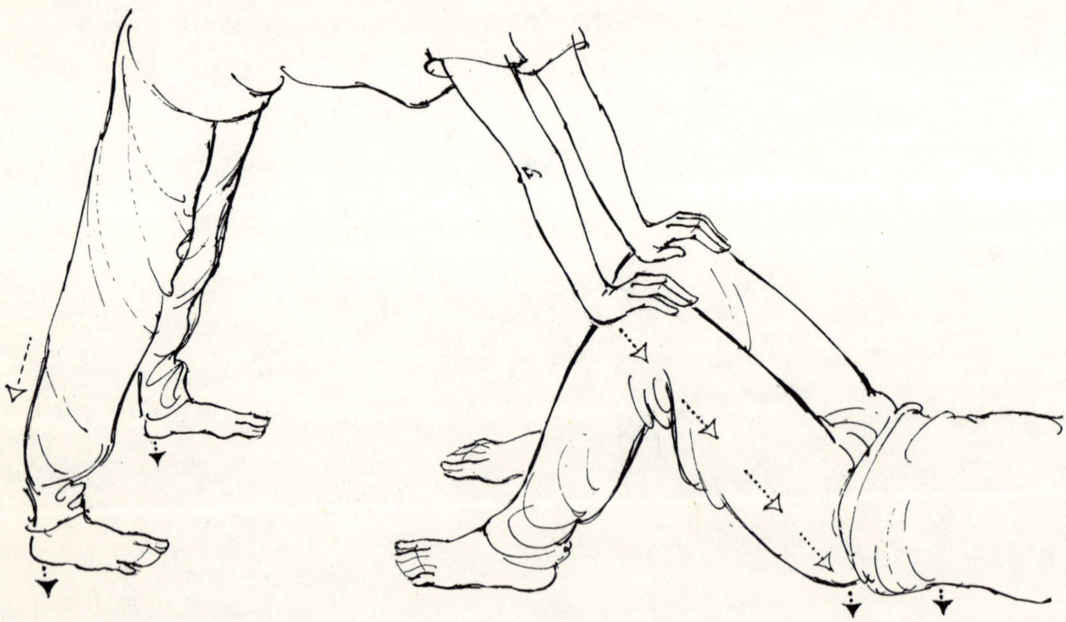

Sacro-Iliac 7

This two-person technique simply "suggests" integrity to the SI joints.

The person on the floor has the feet, ankles, knees and hips all in line and roughly 20 cm apart.

The other person leans through the knees in the direction of the arrows i.e. down through the long axis of the thighs and hips to compress the SI joints against the floor.

Try this for at least 8 breaths.

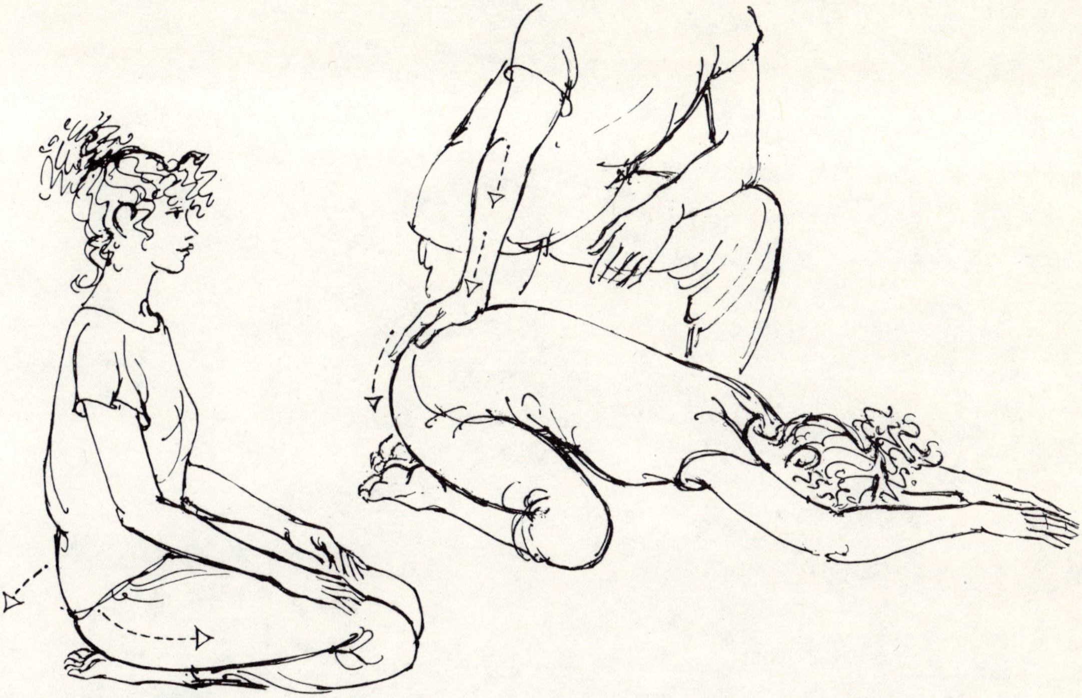

Sacro-Iliac 8

From the start position spread your knees and come forward on to your elbows or stretch your arms completely forward depending on your hip flexibility.

Then use the help of another person leaning centrally through the back of your pelvis in the direction of the arrows.

The pressure should only be increased towards the end of your exhalations. **Do not endure painful resistance of the inner thigh muscles and or the knees.**

Sacro-Iliac 9

As there are only a few specific sacro-iliac techniques, you may have worked through them in one session.

If so finish as you began by relaxing in Sacro-Iliac 1.

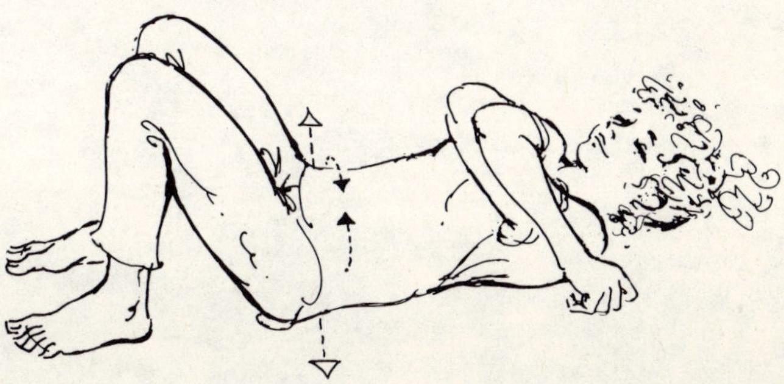

The Upper Structure

The Spine

The spine is the most versatile mechanism in the human structure. Exhaustive studies have been made and much written about the spine and yet it remains, along with the feet, the most misused, abused and vulnerable part of the human framework. Few people have the perfect spine and most can expect to experience some kind of spinal pain or disorder in their lifetime. The spine is the centre to which and from which all energies and forces radiate. It represents the central shaft of the framework: the rest of the structure is an off-shoot of it, the internal organs hang on it, the ribs and breathing apparatus are attached to it, it supports and carries the skull, the spinal cord runs through it and it acts as a scaffolding for the autonomic nervous system. The health of all-important nervous tissue is closely tied to the well-being of the spine. It controls all movement, absorbs all body shocks, has great strength and yet is elastic and flexible. It is a balance mechanism striving to keep body weight balanced with minimum energy expenditure and muscular effort. The spine is constantly dynamic, even during rest and sleep, moving in concert with the breath.

Many people think that the only joints between their vertebrae are where the discs are formed, but there are two more joints between each vertebrae, one on each side. These are the small facet joints and they vary in shape and design in the different regions of the spine. These joints, along with the structure of the vertebrae and the thickness and shape of the discs, determine the nature and degree of spinal movement. The spine's natural versatility is the result of these features combined with its natural curves. It can back-bend, forward-bend, side-bend, twist and combine these movements to form various movement "complexes". For example, a given area of the spine may back-bend, twist and side-bend all at the same time, or one part may forward-bend while another part is back-bending. Movement between each vertebra is relatively small but groups of vertebrae provide considerable ranges of movement as a whole.

Because of the spine's design and its central role in body mechanics, it is particularly prone to stress, rigidity and a large variety of mechanical disturbances. It is vulnerable to all kinds of fixations, strains, sprains and minute traumas, many of which go unnoticed but build up and inevitably lead to early degenerative changes. Shocks to the spine should ideally be kept to a minimum, but forces and stresses are exaggerated when its natural curves are out of balance or rigid in any way. When this occurs shock-absorption and weight-transmission falls on just a few joints instead of being shared through the whole spine and these joints become especially prone to wear and tear. The spine is particularly vulnerable to the force of compression, it can actually buckle and form slight kinks. This

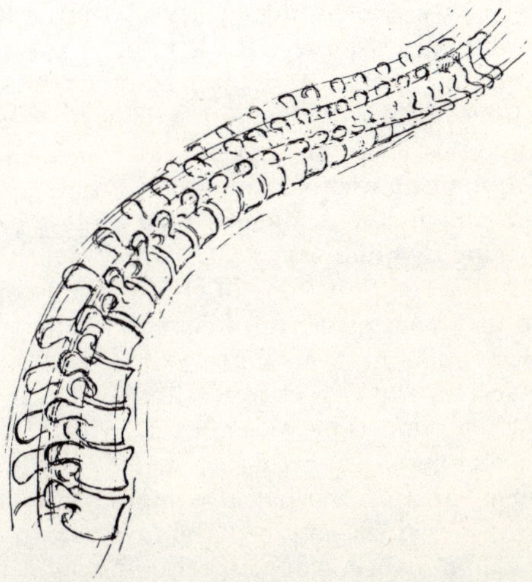

The spine's movements can combine to form movement "complexes"

tendency is exaggerated even more when the spinal muscles shorten, as often happens when extreme physical or psychological effort is anticipated and the body is drawn together as a protective security device. The spine must also adapt to demands and conditions found elsewhere in the body, such as stiffness in the hips, ribs, shoulders, knees, ankles and feet, or any imbalance that disturbs the normal position of the pelvis. Each movement of the body is directly related to the efficiency of its central core, the spinal column. More than any other part of the body the spine craves freedom and balance. This is shown in its potential for flexibility, and its capacity to lengthen and decompress. A well-balanced spine is never rigid: as structure changes it lengthens spontaneously, its mechanism becoming strain-free and more efficient.

Back Pain

Back pain is as prevalent as ever, if not more so. True, we can treat it in a number of ways, but are no closer to making the majority of spines generally healthier. We have to take responsibility for our own back bones if prevention is preferable to treatment. As Wilfred Barlow, the author of *The Alexander Principle*, puts it, "It is primarily a problem of use." Many therapists instruct their patients on how to sit, stand and lift, all valuable in their own way as a kind of prevention, but this leaves patients still feeling like patients: one wrong move and the back may go again. Back pain can be prevented by slowly and progressively changing and balancing structure. Back pain is the culmination of continual poor body mechanics in every day movement and prevention should focus on stretching, releasing, lengthening and balancing the whole spine and the body in general (see page 93 for specific techniques).

Approximately 80% of the world's population experience significant back pain at least once in their lives, and just about everyone can expect to feel tension in their back at one time or another. After heart conditions and arthritis, back disorders come third on the list of complaints which limit physical activity and are the most common cause of occupational disability. The statistics for Britain and the USA alone are staggering. Over 50,000 people a day suffer from backpain and over 20 million working days are lost each year in Britain. As a result 900 million pounds are paid out by social security each year. In the USA 75 million people have back problems and back pain claims at least 7 million new victims each year, of which 5 million are partially disabled and 2 million unable to work at all. Back pain loses 93 million working days each year in the USA and the Americans spend an estimated 5 billion dollars on tests and treatment annually.

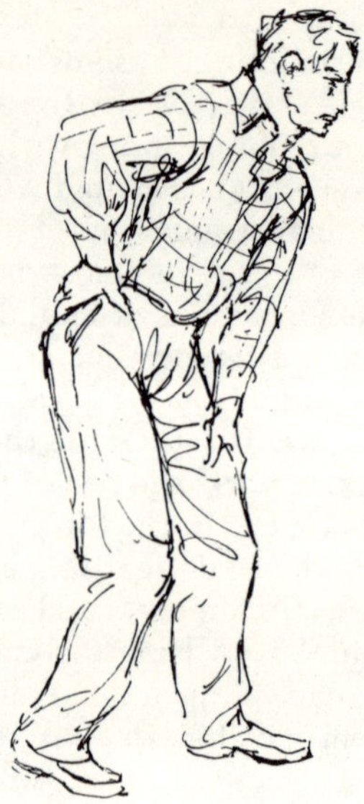

The statistics for Britain and the USA alone are staggering

There can be many contributing factors to back pain: posture, mechanical stresses and strains, degenerative changes, psychological factors, organic problems or diseases of the spine itself. These causes can be further influenced by hereditary factors, injuries, pregnancy, diet and lifestyle in general. But broadly speaking from the structural viewpoint back pain is mainly caused by mechanical strains and degenerative changes in the vertebrae themselves.

High on the list is the postural factor, that is pain related to residual stiffness in the spine which in turn is related to changes in its natural curves. The lower back curve, for example, may be exaggerated, too straight, reversed, side-bent or twisted. The most common of all lower back imbalances is the exaggerated lumbo-sacral angle. This area is most frequently under strain because of all the forces that focus here and this can present a problem to the whole spine. Many imbalances may concentrate on one vertebra in relation to its neighbours. The study of the one bone "out of line" or "fixed" phenomenon has become a science in itself. The so-called osteopathic lesion has probably provoked more literature than any other mechanical fault in the body. But whatever the local mechanics may be, it is necessary to work on the entire spine and the structure as a whole. Any vertebra that gets stuck, hitched, fixed, locked or whatever, indicates that forces within the body are out of balance and have focused on that one vertebra, causing it to buckle under the strain. Very often this situation may resolve with or without treatment but only changing the overall structural pattern will prevent a similar recurrence.

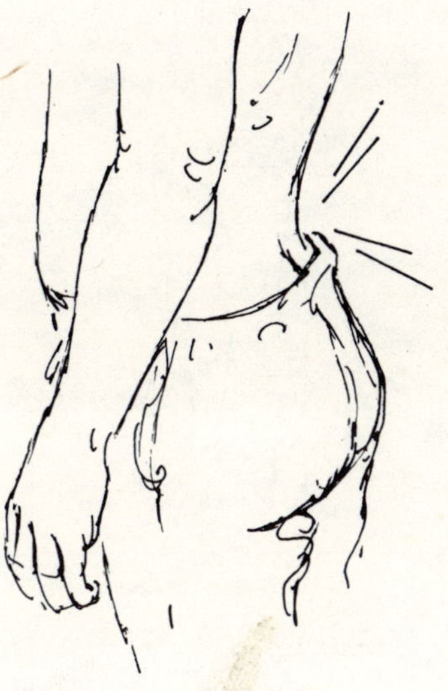

The most common lower back imbalance is the exaggerated lumbo-sacral angle.

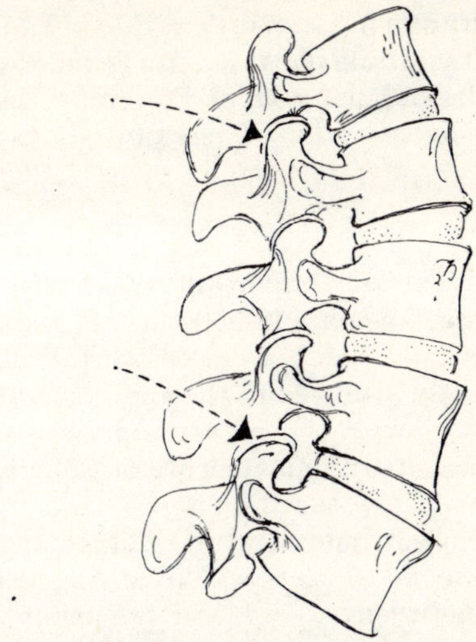

When the spine's natural curves are out of balance, shock absorption falls on a few joints instead of being shared through the whole spine and these joints become especially prone to wear and tear.

Degeneration

The minor joint sprains that build up as a result of daily activity make a major contribution to the degeneration of the spine in general. Small strains and sprains usually repair themselves up to a point but can lead to persistent stiffness if the spine is not loosened, stretched and released regularly. When a spinal joint ceases to work properly, its circulation is affected and this can lead to degenerative and arthritic changes later on and include possible disc problems. Most disc problems are the end result of long-term compression, lack of movement and a drying out of the disc. The shock-absorbing qualities of discs are also seriously impaired by changes in the spinal curves causing body weight to fall on one part of the disc, subsequently thinning and wearing it away. Discs don't slip. They swell, disintegrate, herniate or prolapse but they don't slip. A disc problem is often the end of the line in terms of mechanical abuse. Even though a sudden force may injure the disc, it is likely that strain and degeneration have been developing over a period of time. Luckily only one person in a thousand needs surgery for discs.

People injure their spines doing the simplest things – pulling on a sock, stretching up to a shelf or carrying in the groceries. Some even put their backs out in their sleep, wake up and can't move. But in nearly every case pain in the back cannot be viewed as a local condition; it is accompanied and preceded by imbalances somewhere else in the body. There are forces that push and pull from above and from below, there are forces that grab from behind and drag at the front and so on. Stiffness and imbalance in the legs, hips and shoulders all throw added strain on the spine, and strain in the spine itself can often shift from one level to another. It may not always be possible to change spinal curves radically but by restoring mobility and fluidity, by lengthening and releasing the whole body, we can reduce acute episodes of back pain and minimise the long-term degenerative effects of daily life.

The Ribs

The ribs also play an important role in structural balance and should be kept free, well-adjusted and flexible. They are powerful side levers directly attached to the spine and all but the last few to the breast bone. Slight gliding and twisting movements of the ribs increase and decrease the chest's capacity about 20 times per minute during breathing. It is common to get a "breathing restriction" between two ribs, and the rib joints are common sites for stiffness. Stiffness in the spine may affect the ribs; likewise rib restrictions influence the freedom of the spine itself. Exaggerated spinal curves depress the ribs, they drag at the front, the lower ribs become too close to the pelvis, in turn the upper ribs sag and this leads to the well-known "dowager's hump" at the back of the neck. Sometimes ribs are held too high with the shoulders braced back: this also stiffens the spine, and affects the rest of the structure. When the ribs are free and balanced it usually indicates that the spine is free and the shoulders well supported.

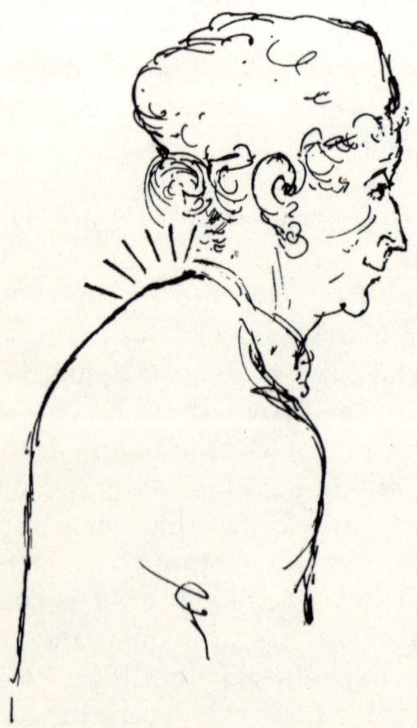

Depressed ribs can lead to the well known "Dowager's Hump" at the base of the neck.

Adjusting the Spine

Most of the spinal techniques also include the ribs as most spinal movement involves the ribs to some extent.

For the spine to adjust effectively, it particularly needs encouragement in lengthening and rotating.

But back-bending, forward and side-bending are also necessary.

Above all the spine needs to be consciously released throughout all the techniques, regardless of the types or ranges of movement suggested or prescribed.

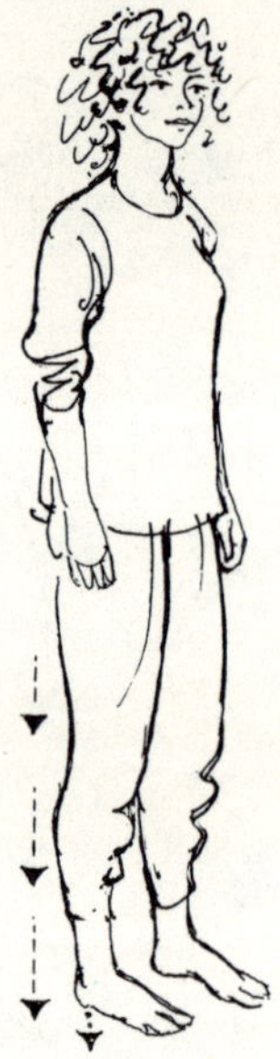

Spine 1

From the SRP exhale down through your heels while feeling particularly heavy in the pelvis.

At the end of each exhalation allow your pelvis to feel at its heaviest and at this point sense your spine release, lengthen and lighten slightly upwards.

Concentrate and release for 6 breaths.

Spine 2

From the previous position simply clasp two fingers gently with your other hand and stretch your arms above your head while maintaining the sense of weight through your pelvis, legs and heels.

Don't arch your back or strain your shoulders upwards.

Feel as if you are hanging from your wrists and each time you exhale soften the skin under your armpits and gently straighten your elbows.

6 to 8 breaths.

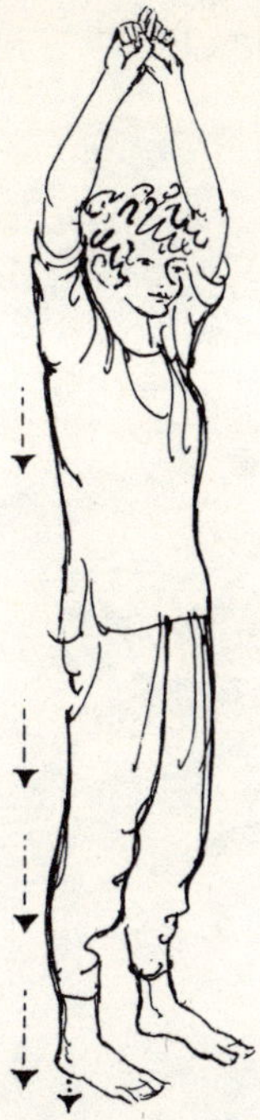

Spine 3

Hanging from a door frame or a bar is useful to decompress the spine.

Have your hands at shoulder width and allow your pelvis to drop by bending your knees.

Keep your feet lightly on the floor.

Allow your pelvis and legs to feel particularly heavy towards the end of each exhalation.

Stretch in this way for 4 breaths.

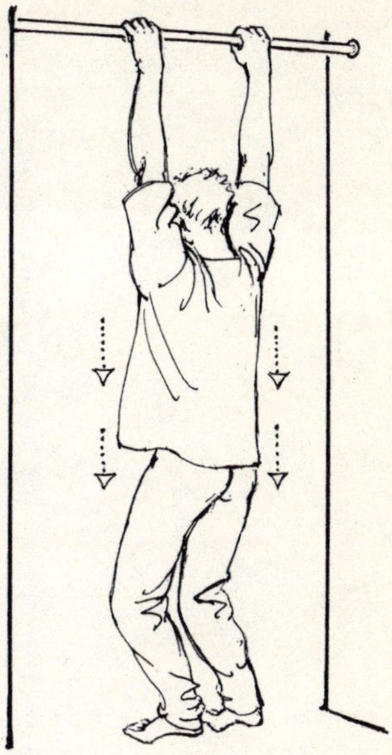

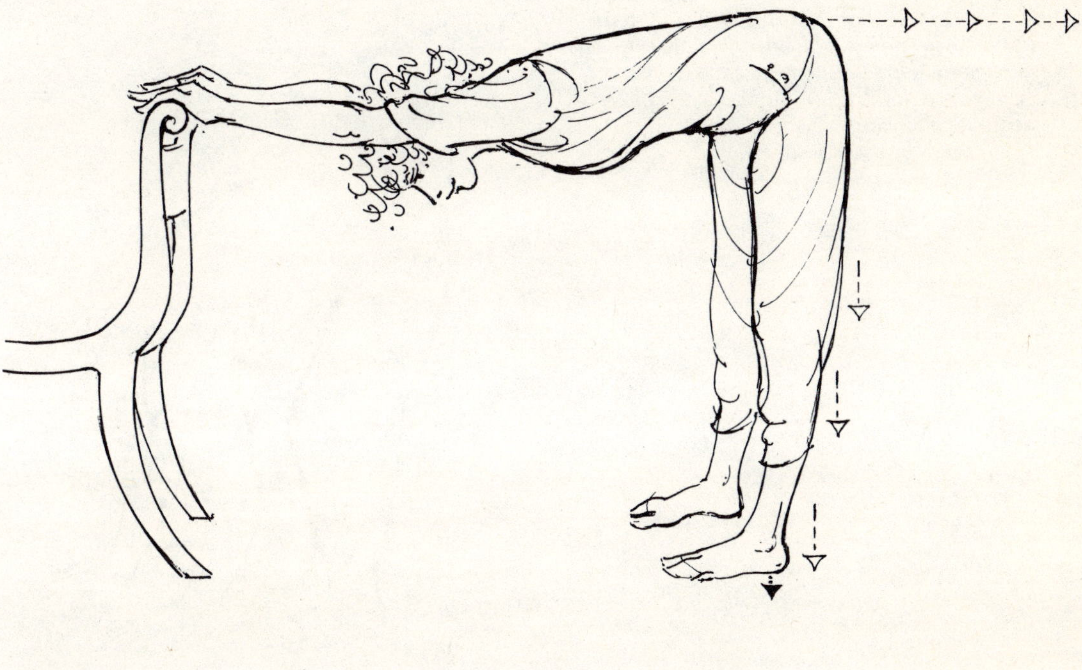

Spine 4

Lengthen your spine away from a table, ledge or chair.

Ideally your trunk and legs should form a right angle, ankles directly under your hips. (You can check this out by using a mirror.)

Towards the end of each exhalation release between your shoulder blades and project your tail bone backwards in order to lengthen your lower back and separate the vertebrae.

Don't arch your lower back by projecting your tail bone upwards—but try to keep your tail bone projection through a horizontal plane.

Lengthen for 6 exhalations.

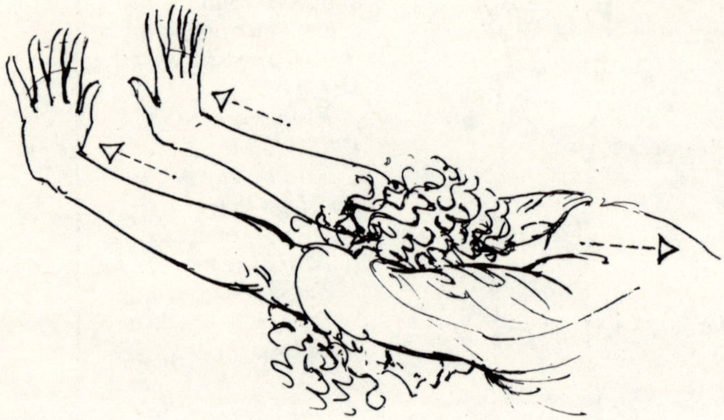

Spine 5

An alternative way to use the previous technique is against a wall. The instruction is the same except that pushing on a wall with your fingers spread wide gives an added leverage to help lengthen the spine.

Study the illustration for the correct positioning of your arms and hands.

Lengthen for 6 exhalations.

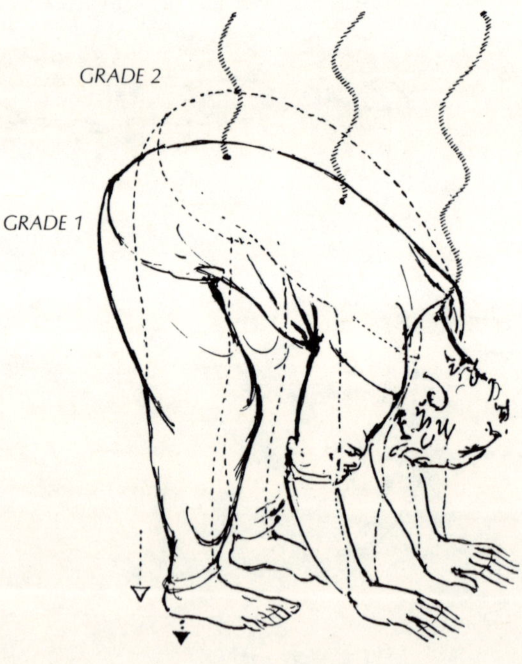

Spine 6

Basic forward bending from the SRP can also be used to release and lengthen the spine.

Grade 1 involves bending the knees; if your legs are supple enough try keeping the knees straight as in Grade 2.

In each case allow the spine to lengthen during each exhalation.

Think broad across the back of the pelvis.

At the end of each exhalation imagine you are a puppet that has had its strings cut and allow the head and shoulders to drop softly.

Work and release for at least 6 breaths and come up slowly, exhaling.

Spine 7

This technique, used in Hips 4, can also be used to release the spine.

The instruction is the same but concentrate more on lengthening the spine downwards towards the floor.

Be particularly aware of the foot position as shown in the illustration and explained in Hips 4.

Feel most of your weight through your back heel.

Imagine your tail bone is being pulled downwards towards your back heel and your spine releasing outwards and downwards, to the side.

Don't let the upper shoulder drop forward; keep it back and open.

Work for at least 6 breaths and come up slowly, exhaling. Repeat on the other side.

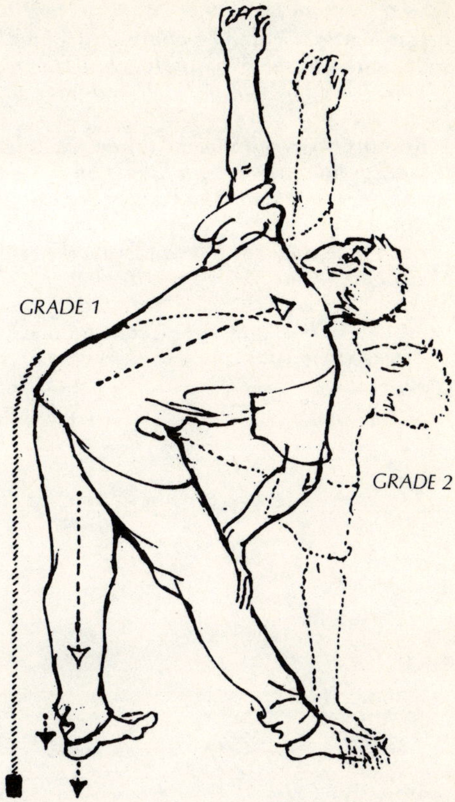

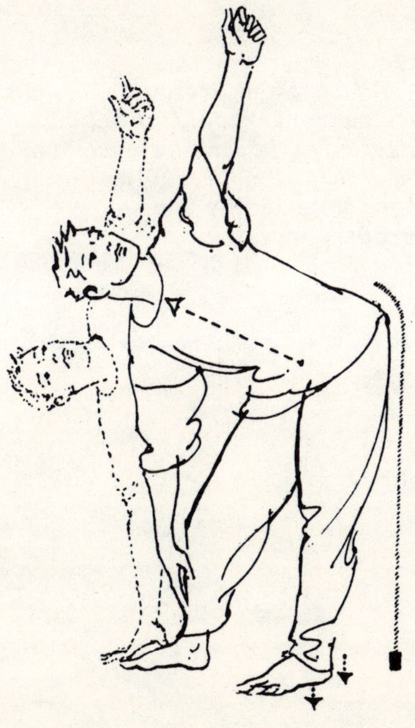

Spine 8

Exactly the same procedure as Spine 7 except the front leg is slightly bent.

Bending the front knee gives a slightly different sense of release in the spine and allows it to side-bend and hang a little lower.

6 breaths. Come up slowly, exhaling, and repeat on the other side.

Spine 9

Sit side on to a wall on a chair or stool with your inner shoulder lightly touching the wall.

Your feet should be parallel and flat on the floor.

Keeping your pelvis as heavy as possible, twist around and put both hands on the wall at shoulder height and just wider than shoulder width.

Each time you exhale, exaggerate the rotation by dropping your pelvis into the chair, releasing between the shoulder blades and using the wall as a lever to rotate against.

Release and rotate for 4 to 6 breaths and change sides.

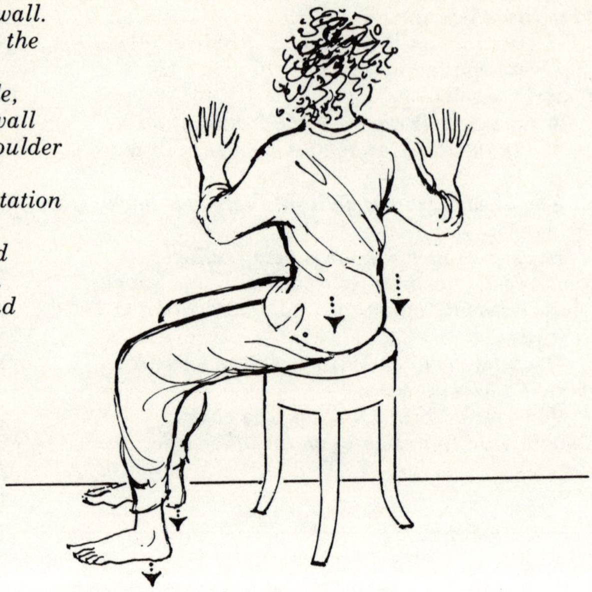

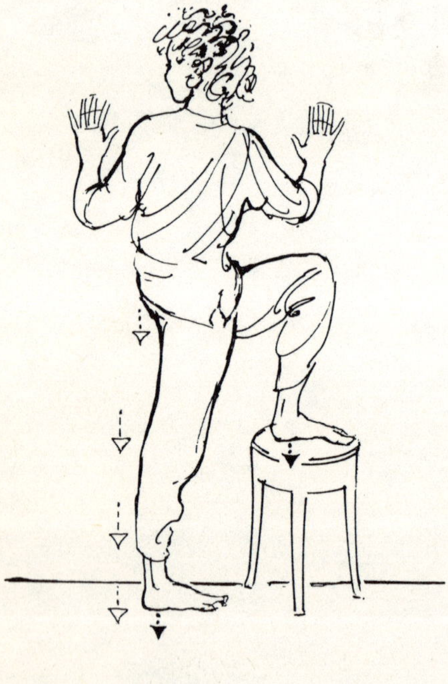

Spine 10

A variation of Spine 9 is to stand with inner leg on the stool, inner shoulder touching the wall and rotating in the same way, except that as you exhale drop the weight from your pelvis down through your standing heel.

4 breaths each side.

Spine 11

This technique puts quite a strong side-bending stretch on to the spine. Note that:

- *the pelvis is resting on the wall.*
- *the inside foot is about 30 cm from the wall.*
- *the outside knee is bent.*
- *the outside heel is raised.*

Control the side-bending with your outer arm on your hip or leg. Release the spine sideways as you exhale, sliding your upper hand downwards each time.

To give your lower back a sense of security in this technique, continually push your inside foot firmly downward into the floor and keep your tail bone dropped.

Release slowly for 4 breaths on each side.

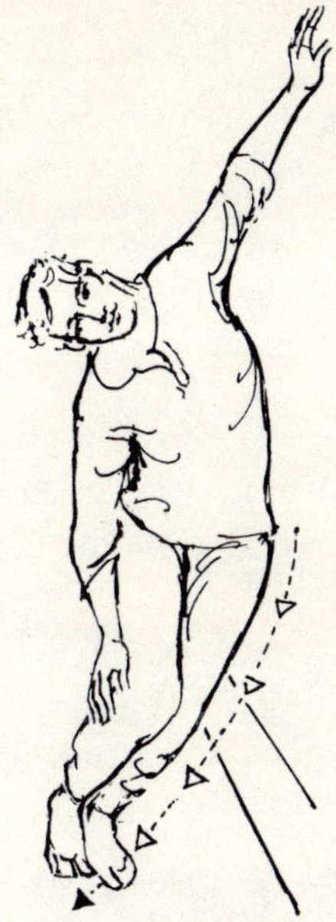

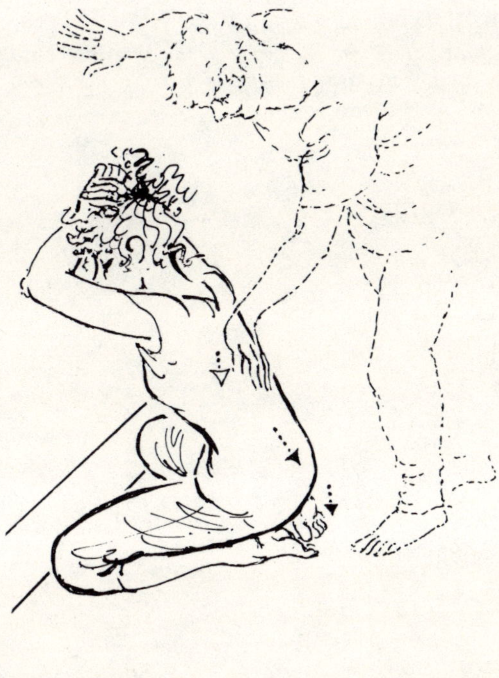

Spine 12

This technique is useful for releasing the upper back. Sit on a cushion if your knees and ankles feel discomfort. Your knees should be touching the wall with your buttocks on your heels.

Rest your forehead on your hands.

Each time you exhale push your pelvis downwards and direct your chest on to the wall, consciously releasing between your shoulder blades as you do so.

Someone can help you by leaning from above and working gently down your upper back step by step as you exhale. The heel of the hand should be used and pressure should fall exactly central to each vertebra. This is strictly an upper and middle back technique: your partner should stop before reaching the lower back.

Work for as many breaths you feel appropriate, 8 breaths is normally maximum for a good response.

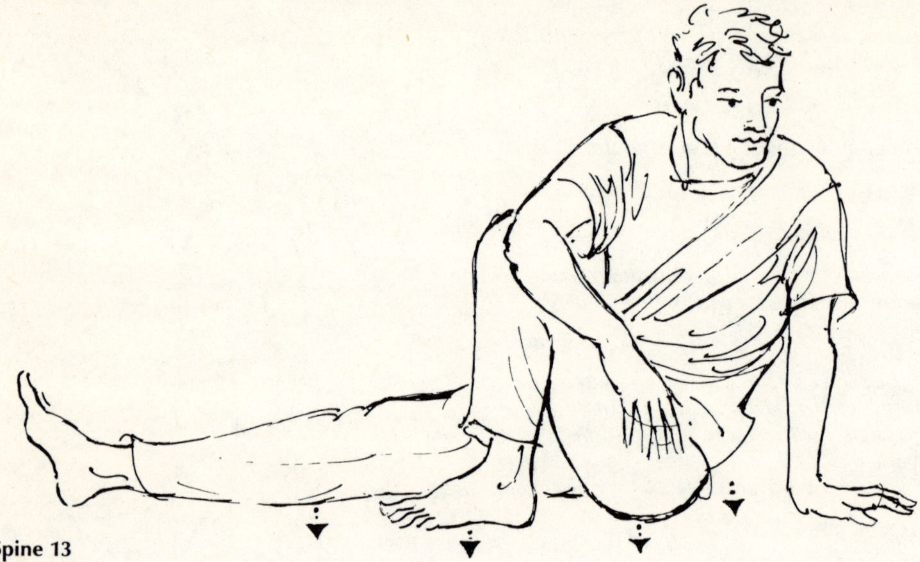

Spine 13

This simple sitting twist involves keeping both buttocks on the floor and giving adequate support with the outstretched arm.

You are twisting across your bent leg using the back of your arm as a lever.

Each time you exhale feel heavy in your pelvis, release between the shoulder blades, slightly lengthen your spine and rotate a little further towards the end of your exhalation.

4 to 6 breaths and change sides.

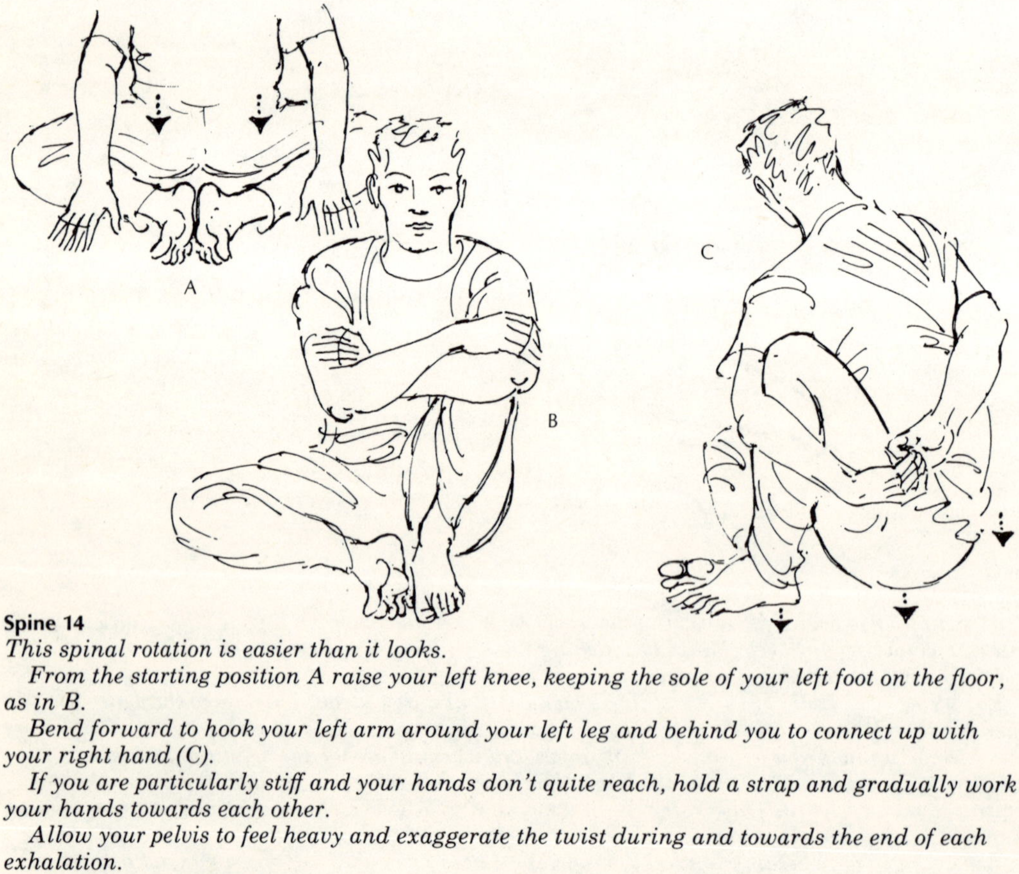

Spine 14

This spinal rotation is easier than it looks.

From the starting position A raise your left knee, keeping the sole of your left foot on the floor, as in B.

Bend forward to hook your left arm around your left leg and behind you to connect up with your right hand (C).

If you are particularly stiff and your hands don't quite reach, hold a strap and gradually work your hands towards each other.

Allow your pelvis to feel heavy and exaggerate the twist during and towards the end of each exhalation.

6 breaths and change sides.

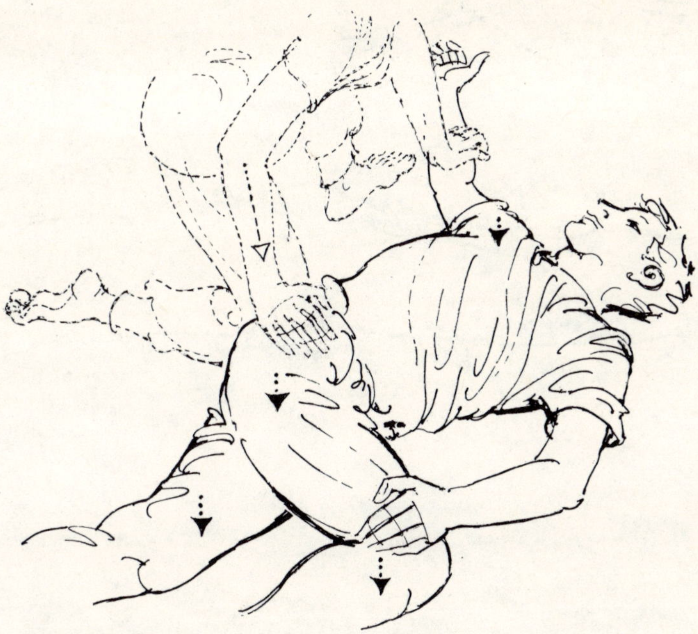

Spine 15

This floor rotation is particularly good for the spine even though you have to break through stiffness in the shoulders for the spine to get the full benefit.

Cross your right knee over your left and lower your right knee down towards your left side and fix it to the floor with your left hand.

Stretch your right arm out to a 45° angle behind you.

Each time you exhale, feel heavy in the pelvis, fix the knee to the floor more firmly and allow your outstretched arm to drop and settle in order to increase the rotation of your spine.

Another person can assist by fixing your knee or pelvis and directing the outstretched arm downwards.

Don't force it, but produce a strong enough sensation of stretch to bite on so that you have enough to release from.

6 breaths each side should be ample.

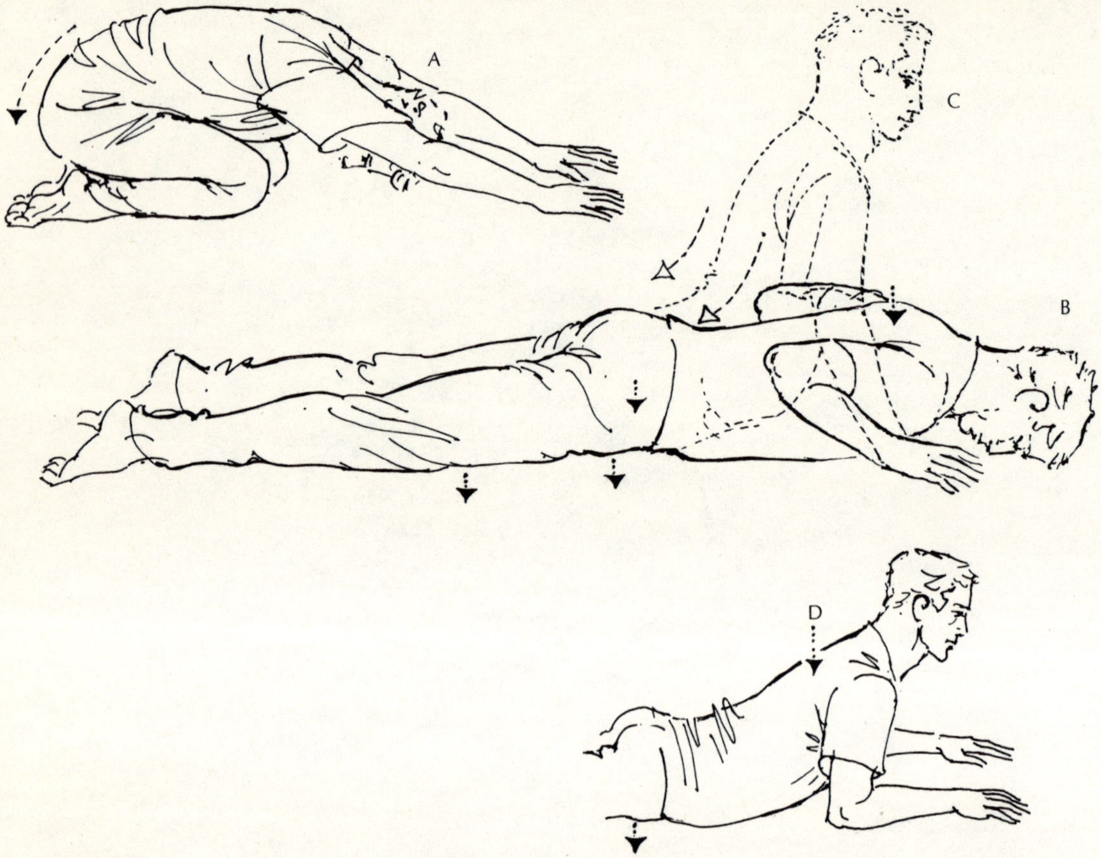

Spine 16

This is the only true back-bending technique in the book because most back bends need personal instruction to get them "right" without undue strain.

This technique, however, is easy and beneficial.

From the starting position A, stretch out your arms with your palms face down and at shoulder width, fingers spread wide and pointing forwards.

Then, keeping your chest close to the floor, move into position B: elbows facing upwards, fingertips roughly under your collar bones.

Lie still for a few breaths and concentrate on widening across the back of your pelvis and consciously releasing between your shoulder blades.

Exhale down through the palms of your hands a few times and when you feel ready, slowly push up to straighten your arms as you exhale. The important points are:

- *keep your shoulders down away from your ears.*
- *keep your pubic bone on the floor.*
- *keep relaxed and broad across the lower back and pelvis.*
- *keep consciously releasing and relaxing between your shoulder blades and projecting your chest slightly forwards.*

The lower back should not be forced upwards into a back bend, but should drop downwards away from your chest during the exhalation.

Work and release for at least 6 breaths and come down slowly. If you feel any discomfort in the lower back, or feel exceptionally stiff during this technique use the bent-elbow variation as in D, until you feel ready to straighten your arms.

Spine 17

This is a similar technique to Ankles 7, but is used to stretch the spine in forward bending.

With your heels slightly raised on a towel or cushion, squat down, keeping your feet together and your heels on your towel.

Open your knees as wide as you can without lifting the inner arch of your feet excessively.

Place your trunk between your knees. Stay heavy in the pelvis, project your tail bone down to your heels, dropping your shoulders and elbows each time you exhale.

Eventually Grade 2 will become possible i.e. without a support.

Work and release for about 8 breaths.

The idea is to open up the whole of the spine.

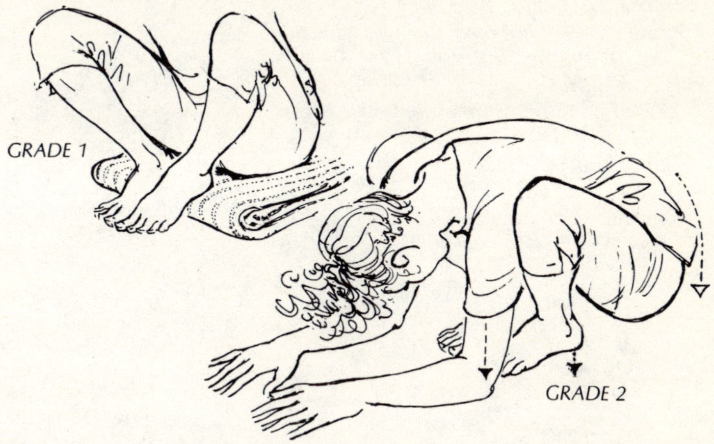

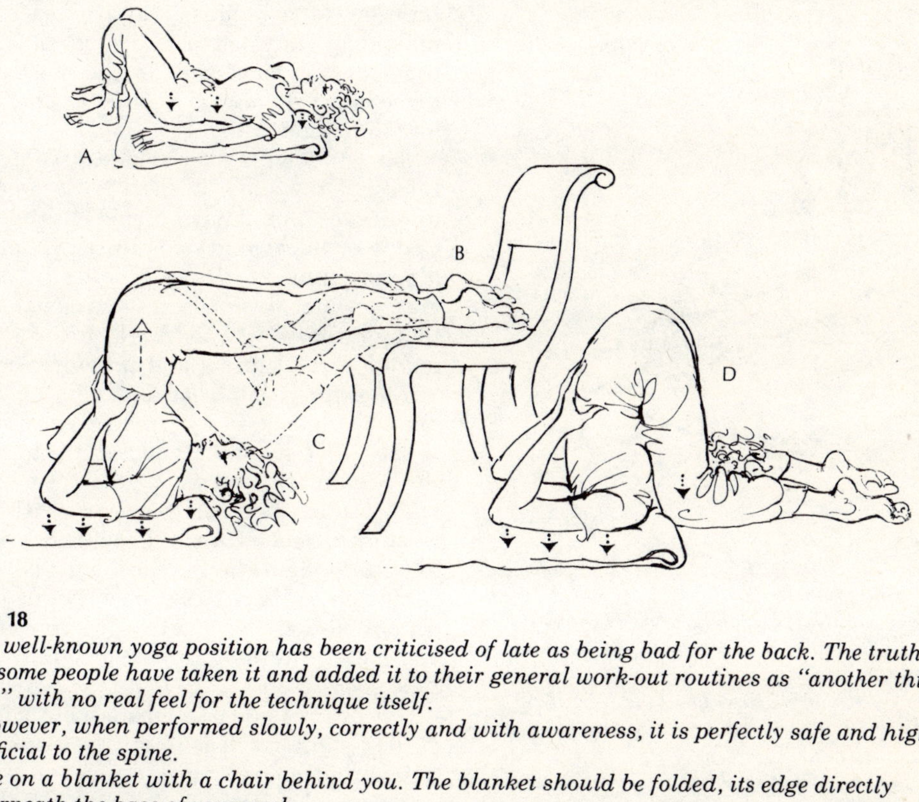

Spine 18

This well-known yoga position has been criticised of late as being bad for the back. The truth is that some people have taken it and added it to their general work-out routines as "another thing to do" with no real feel for the technique itself.

However, when performed slowly, correctly and with awareness, it is perfectly safe and highly beneficial to the spine.

Lie on a blanket with a chair behind you. The blanket should be folded, its edge directly underneath the base of your neck.

Lengthen the back of your neck, feel broad across your upper back and take a few breaths.

When you feel ready, exhale as you push down with your hands and take your feet over your head and put them on the chair.

Support your back with your hands, keeping your elbows as close together as possible.

Keep your head central, chin into chest.

Exhale down through your elbows, shoulders and neck, consciously releasing areas of tension as you do so.

If the knee-straight position is comfortable as in B, start to bend your knees as in C.

Then gradually lower the knees and dispense with the chair when you feel ready.

The final stage may take some time to cultivate. Don't rush it and don't overstretch your back, just slowly and gradually release it.

Start with 5 or 6 breaths and eventually build up to 15 or 20.

Spine 19

In the LRP, imagine your spine broadening and lengthening for its entire length as you exhale. Visualise your spinal muscles separating away from the spine, and your tail bone and the crown of your head lengthening away from each other.

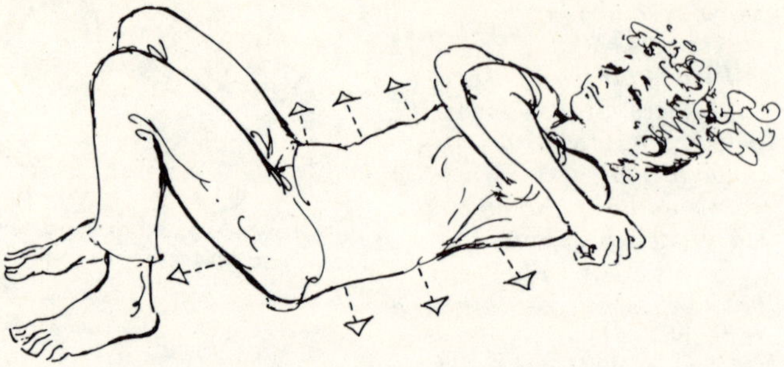

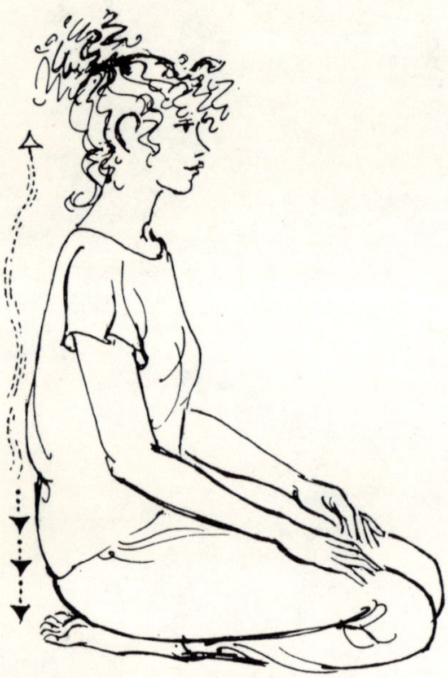

Spine 20

Sit on your heels with your knees together and your hands in your lap.

Close your eyes and drop your chin very slightly downwards to lengthen the back of your neck.

Sense each of your exhalations travelling down your back into your pelvis which becomes heavier.

At the end of each exhalation, sense your pelvis at its heaviest, at which point and before you breathe in, your spine spontaneously lightens and lengthens slightly upwards.

Practise for at least 15 breaths.

The value of this very subtle technique should not be underestimated. When performed properly, its effect on the spine is quite remarkable.

Backpain Techniques

The problem of back pain is so extensive that it is impossible to include in a book specific tailor-made techniques that exactly fit each individual imbalance. This is not even necessary as back pain in the mechanical sense is nearly always related to poor body mechanics generally.

The following techniques emphasise releasing the spine itself. They are gentle, low-grade techniques aimed initially at easing and decompressing the spine and are a preparation for the techniques involving greater ranges of voluntary movement. Even though these specific back release techniques ease stiffness and provide a means of relief for painful backs, we still need to approach backpain wholistically i.e. attend to the whole structure and not just to where the symptoms appear.

Therefore become familiar with and master the feel of this routine. It is suitable for all configurations of back imbalances. After four to six weeks start working on the general non-graded and low-graded routines and build into the intermediate routines as time goes by.

However, if you are a back pain sufferer of long standing, it is worth referring back to this routine from time to time.

A 4-week back release programme for back pain

Week 1 DAILY

Start in SRP
Pelvis 1
Pelvis 2, 3 or 4
Pelvis 5
Pelvis 8
Sacro-iliac 7
Finish in LRP

Week 2 DAILY

Start in SRP
Pelvis 2, 3 or 4
Spine 1
Spine 4
Spine 9
Hips 8
Pelvis 7 grades 1 & 2 only
Hips 24
Sacro-iliac 8
Hips 31
Finish in LRP

Week 3 DAILY

Start in LRP
Hips 8
Sacro-iliac 2
Sacro-iliac 4
Spine 15
Hips 24
Sacro-iliac 8
Spine 4
Spine 7
Spine 8
Pelvis 2, 3 or 4
Finish in LRP

Week 4 DAILY

Start in SRP
Pelvis 2, 3 or 4
Hips 3 grade 1 & 2
LRP
Hips 8
Hips 11 grade 1 or 2
Hips 12 grade 1
Spine 15
Hips 24
Pelvis 6
Sacro-iliac 4
Spine 9
Sacro-iliac 3
Spine 20
Hips 31

The Shoulders

Excessive tightness in the shoulders is extremely common. They are a frequent site of misuse since they are involved in so much daily activity and so much emotional tension is invested in them. It is even common to see professional athletes with tight, badly balanced shoulders, and there is a staggering number of people running, circuit training, swimming, playing tennis or squash and doing all kinds of class work with tight, "held" and fixed shoulders. It seems that nowhere in the body is the concept of balance and freedom more misunderstood than in the shoulders.

The shoulder girdle includes the collar bone, the shoulder blade and the top of the arm which fits into the shoulder blade to form the actual shoulder joint. It is a ball-and-socket joint like the hip but much shallower, less stable and more mobile. In fact by nature the shoulder is the most mobile joint in the whole body. The girdle forms a yoke hung across the top of the rib cage and its only connection to the spine is through the collar bone and breast bone which in turn connect to the spine via the ribs. The shoulder girdle supports no weight except for the hanging arms and is itself supported by muscles from the head and neck, and by the spine via the breast bone and ribs. This design allows the arms to move freely without putting pressure on the upper chest where the heart and lungs are situated.

The shoulder girdle is particularly vulnerable to structural stiffness and imbalance because of its lightness and its great potential for movement. Freedom and balance of the shoulders is vital to overall balance. Nearly every bone in the trunk from the base of the skull to the pelvis provides some kind of attachment for muscles also attached to the shoulder girdle. These muscles extend in all directions, to the head, around the rib cage from the spine, through the entire length of the back; they are attached to every vertebra from the top of the neck to the back of the pelvis, and to the front of the belly.

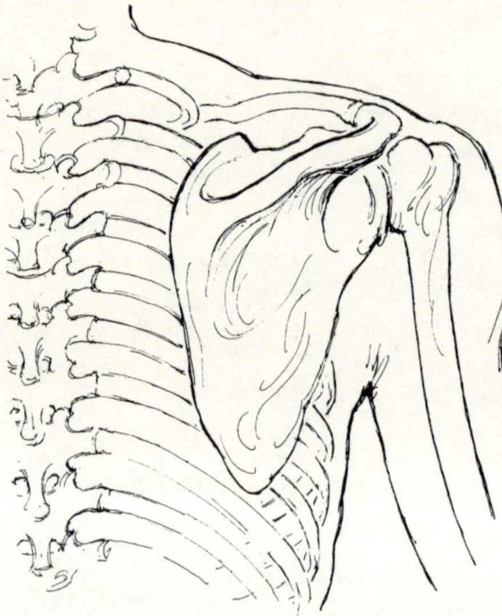

It seems that nowhere in the body is the concept of balance and freedom more misunderstood and underestimated than in the shoulders.

When the arm moves, the whole shoulder girdle has to move in harmony, but harmony is only possible when the ball and socket joint itself is kept free for action. The ramifications of tight shoulders are extensive: restricted shoulders affect rib freedom in breathing, reduce movement of the arms, stiffen the neck, affect head balance and the balance of the entire spine, leading to upper or lower back pain, cause tension in the hands and wrists and generally distort the balance of the structure *en masse*.

Loosening the Shoulders

The first three shoulder techniques use mainly visualisation and are ideal for preparing the shoulders for the remainder of the techniques.

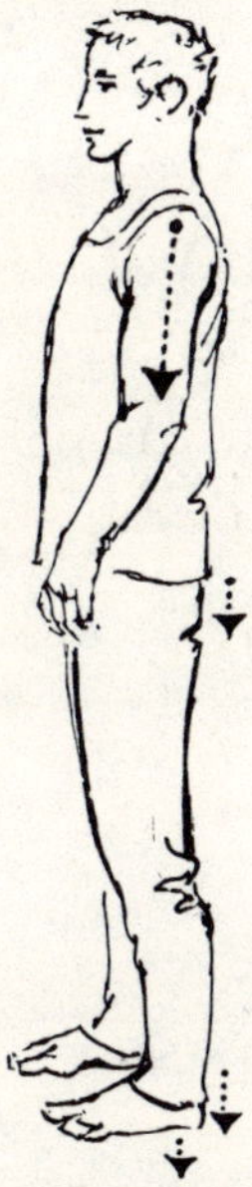

Shoulders 1

From the SRP visualise the arms as being very heavy from your wrists.

Imagine your arms connected to your shoulders by two thick pieces of elastic that are pulled and stretched downwards with each exhalation.

Each time you exhale the weight of the arms stretches the elastic more and more.

Release and visualise for at least 6 breaths.

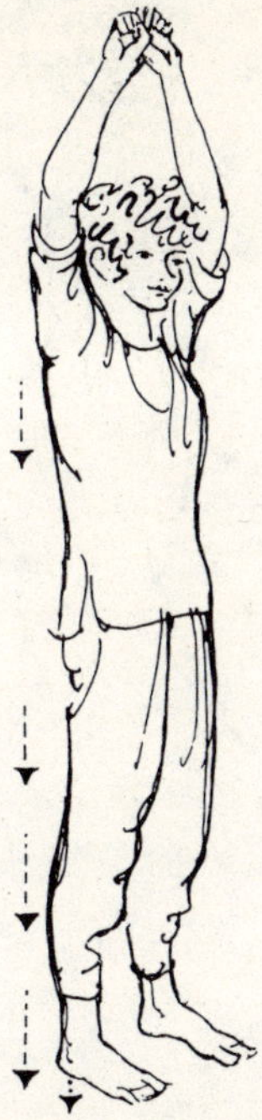

Shoulders 2

From the SRP and feeling particularly heavy down through your pelvis and heels, softly clasp two fingers of one hand with the other hand and stretch above your head.

The shoulders stay down, only the arms raise as you gently straighten your elbows.

Imagine the skin underneath your arms and in front of your elbows softening each time you exhale down through your spine, pelvis and legs through your feet into the floor.

Hold and release for at least 8 breaths.

Shoulders 3

Simply sitting with your feet flat on the floor, have your hands at shoulder width on a table or desk in front of you.

Keeping your knees at a right angle and with your back in a neutral position i.e. neither too straight nor too bent, visualise the following as you exhale:

- *pelvis dropping*
- *neck lengthening*
- *two imaginary lines extending sideways from the tips of your shoulders that gradually get longer and longer.*

Visualise for at least 8 breaths.

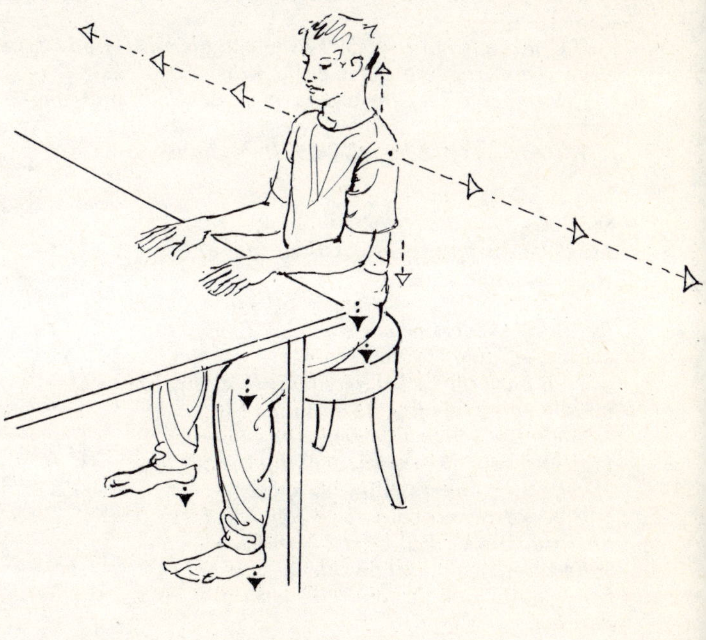

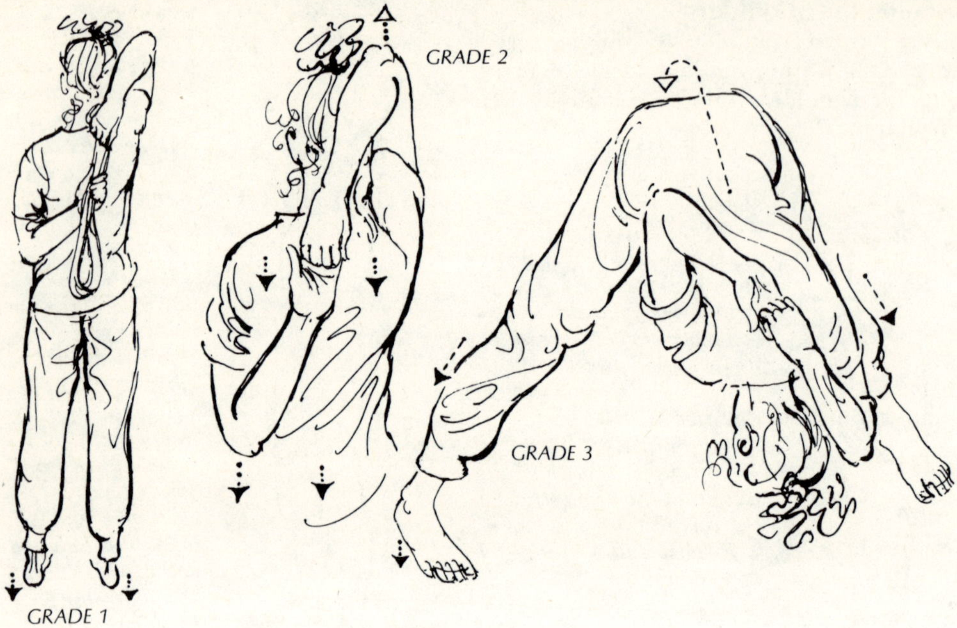

Shoulders 4

Take a few breaths standing in the release position to relax your shoulders and then link your hands as shown in the illustration. Try not to arch your back as you do so by maintaining the sense of the tail bone dropping down to the floor.

If your hands don't reach each other you can use a strap or belt as in Grade 1.

Each time you exhale allow your shoulders to release and relax without losing the grip on your hands.

If Grade 2 is relatively easy you can also use Grade 3, incorporating the legs-apart forward bend. This exaggerates the pull on the shoulders.

Remember to keep the toes turned slightly in and lengthen your spine downwards during each exhalation.

Work from 4 to 8 breaths and then change arms.

Shoulders 5

Many people find this difficult at first due to stiffness in the wrists.

From the SRP take a few breaths to relax and free the shoulders before you even attempt to slide your hands up your back.

First push the little fingers together, then the middle and index fingers and then the thumbs.

Each time you exhale draw the elbows back to stretch your shoulders, pushing the borders of your little fingers into your spine.

Don't arch your back, keep your tail bone dropped. Work for at least 6 breaths.

Eventually you will be able to place your hands quite high up your back with your palms together.

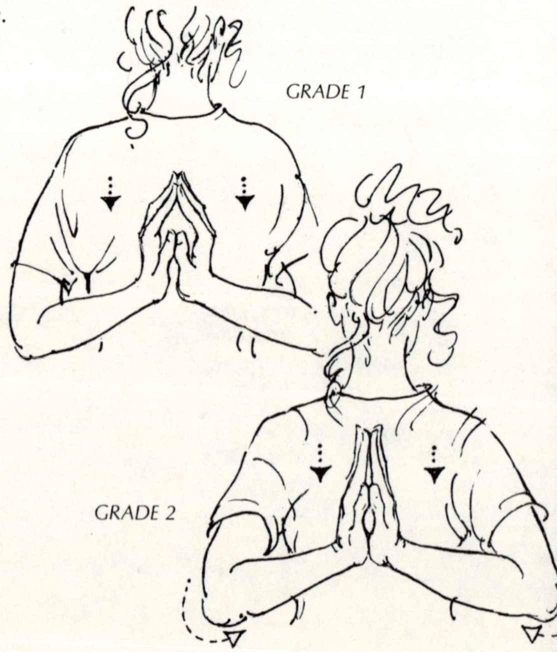

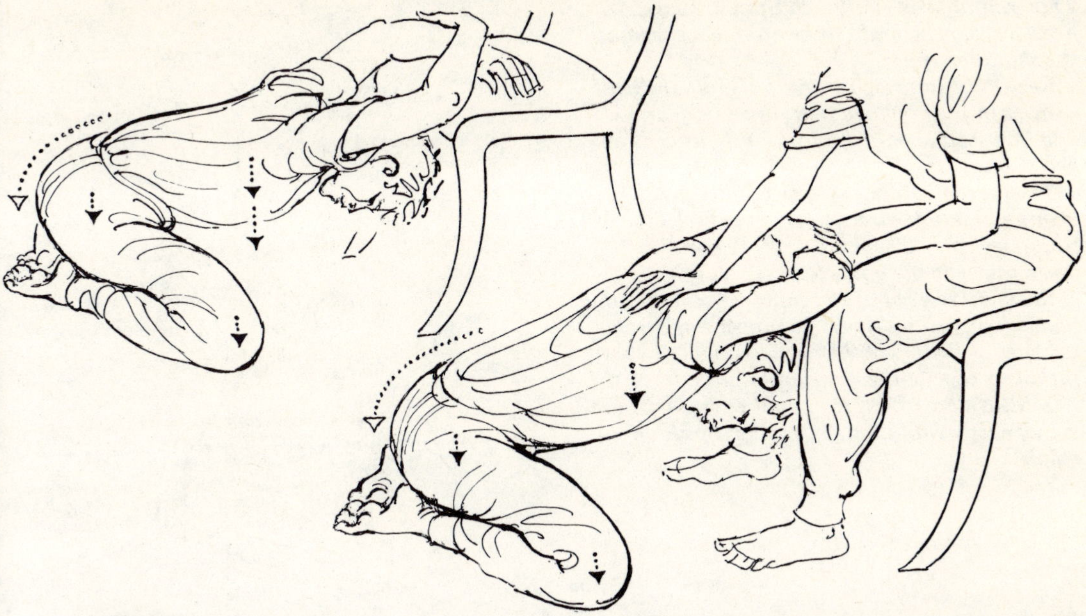

Shoulders 6
Cross your arms over the edge of a chair, drop your head through and allow your chest to feel heavy.

Keep your knees wide and your pelvis back on your heels. Release and relax your shoulders each time you exhale.

You can do the same thing on someone's knees while he or she pushes gently down between or on your shoulder blades, to exaggerate the stretch.

The pressure should be directed in line with the arrows. 6 to 8 breaths.

Shoulders 7
Knees wide.

Buttocks on heels.

Stretch your arms up the wall at an angle of roughly 45° to the floor.

Keep your hands at shoulder width and your fingers spread wide.

Each time you exhale allow your chest to drop without sliding your hands down the wall.

If you are tight in the shoulders you may not be able to straighten your elbows completely (Grade 1).

Push on the wall to keep your elbows as straight as possible.

This can provide a strong stretch in the shoulders and for some people the Grade 2 range of movement takes a long time to achieve.

Soften and release your shoulders for 6 to 8 breaths.

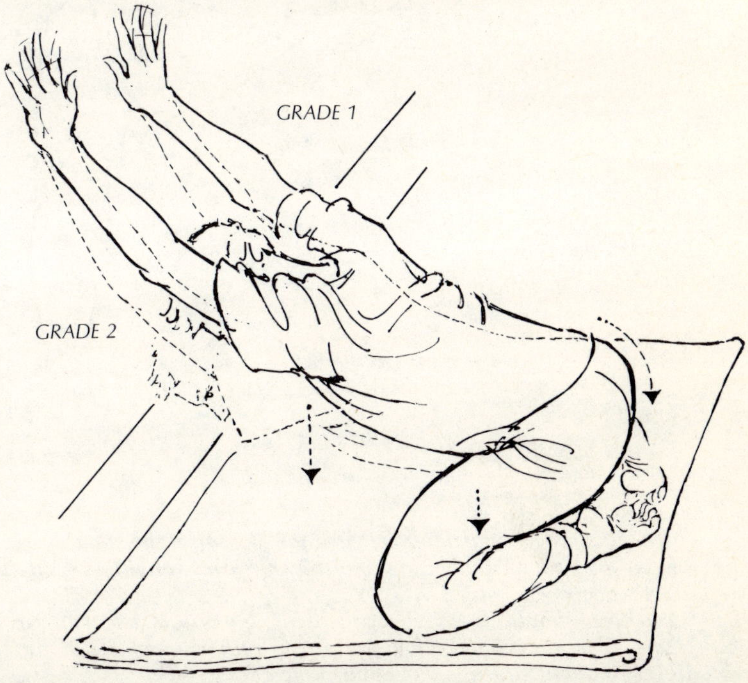

Shoulders 8

This technique is similar to Spine 12 except the arms are kept straight to localise movement at the shoulder joints.

Keep your knees wide and well into the wall and, as in the previous technique, keep arms and hands at shoulder width and buttocks on heels.

The person helping simply applies gentle leaning pressure directly on to the vertebrae of the upper back. The fingertips are pointing down towards the buttocks, the soft fleshy heel of the hand is used as the contact point and the hand slowly slides down the upper back from the base or bottom of the neck to no lower than the lower edge of the shoulder blades.

A little more pressure is applied towards the end of each exhalation. 6 breaths should be ample.

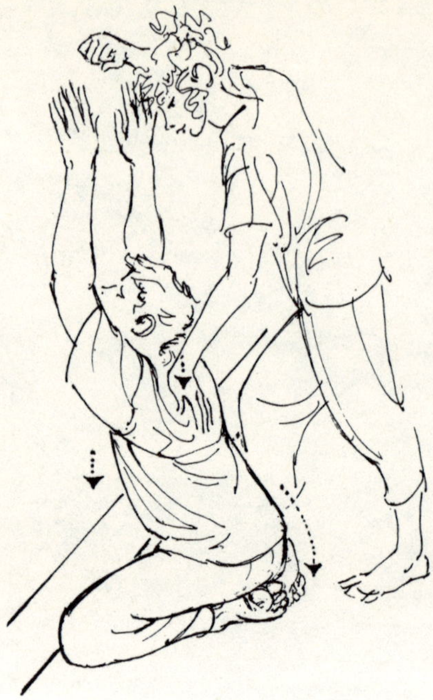

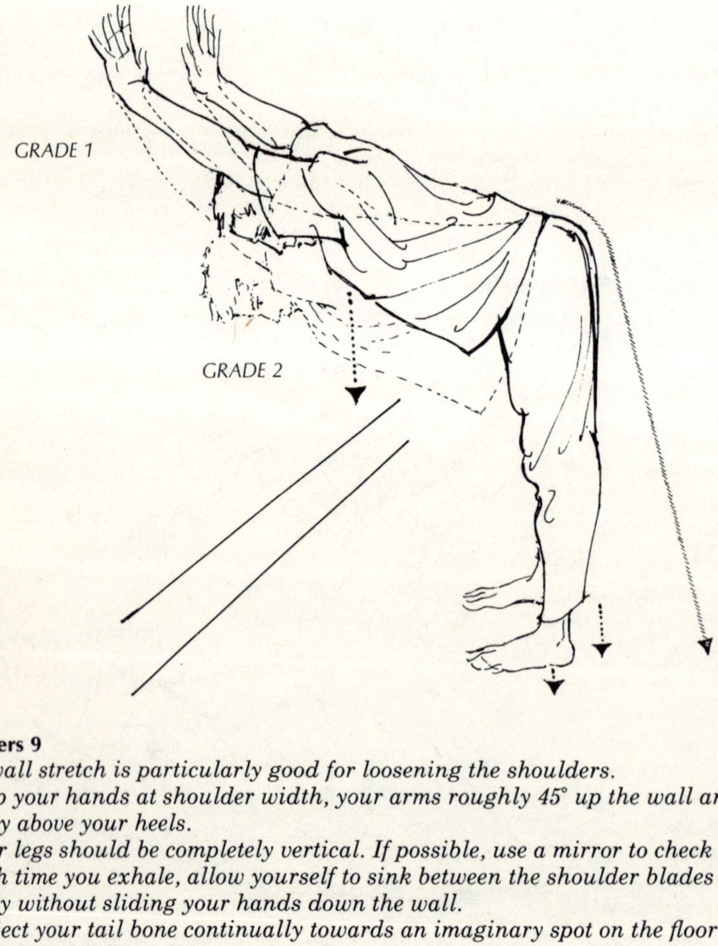

Shoulders 9

This wall stretch is particularly good for loosening the shoulders.

Keep your hands at shoulder width, your arms roughly 45° up the wall and your tail bone directly above your heels.

Your legs should be completely vertical. If possible, use a mirror to check this.

Each time you exhale, allow yourself to sink between the shoulder blades and drop your chest slightly without sliding your hands down the wall.

Project your tail bone continually towards an imaginary spot on the floor behind you.

4 to 8 breaths depending on your tolerance.

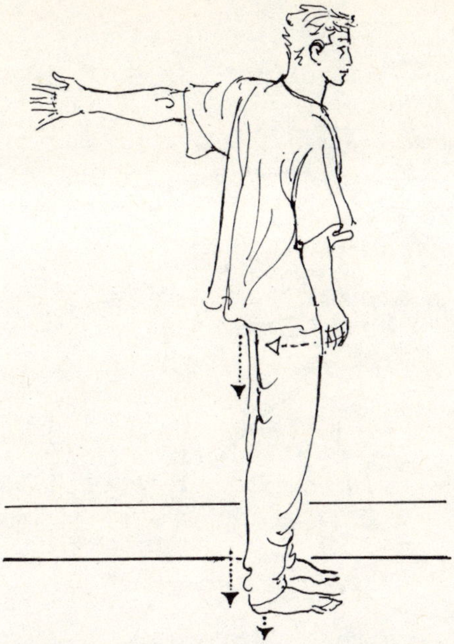

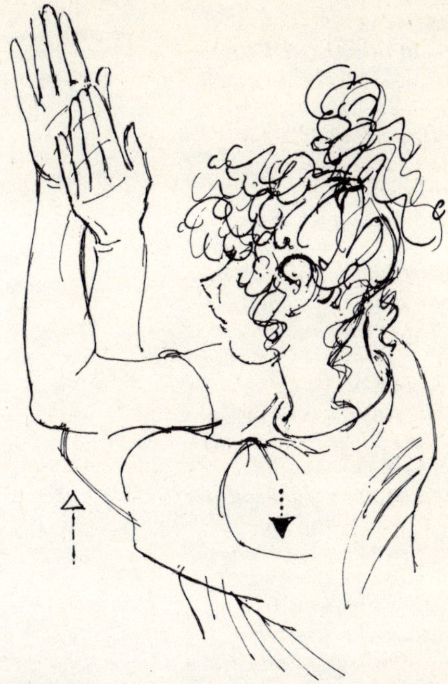

Shoulders 10

The shoulder closer to the wall is released by leaning into the wall and turning slightly away from it.

Your feet should be no more than a few centimetres from the wall.

Keep a sense of your tail bone dropping.

Exaggerate the stretch towards the end of each exhalation.

Work for 6 breaths and change sides.

Shoulders 11

To open the space between the shoulder blades, cross your elbows in front of you and push your palms together.

The hand of the upper arm will inevitably be higher than the other.

Each time you exhale raise your arms slightly upwards without lifting your shoulders.

Open and release for 6 exhalations.

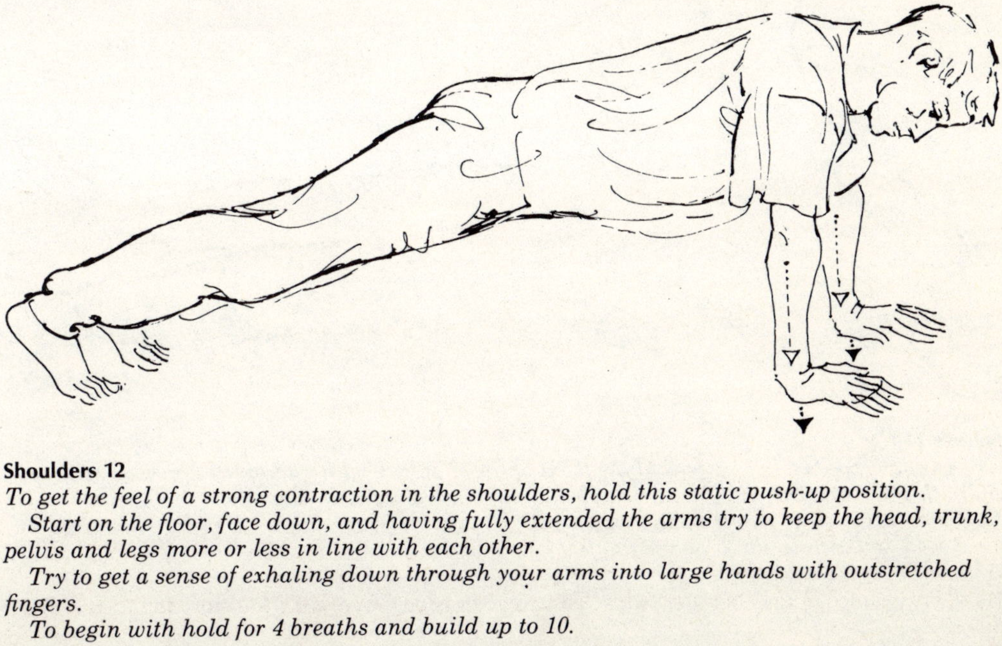

Shoulders 12

To get the feel of a strong contraction in the shoulders, hold this static push-up position.

Start on the floor, face down, and having fully extended the arms try to keep the head, trunk, pelvis and legs more or less in line with each other.

Try to get a sense of exhaling down through your arms into large hands with outstretched fingers.

To begin with hold for 4 breaths and build up to 10.

Shoulders 13

Some of the assisted stretch-and-release techniques are very much like manipulations. This is particularly true of this technique.

A folded towel or pad is placed between the knee of the helper and the spine of the person being stretched.

The knee should be directly in the mid-line.

The person being stretched has the fingers interlocked at the back of the head or neck.

The elbows are slowly pulled back against counter-pressure with the knee towards the end of each exhalation.

This is a powerful technique that stretches the pectoral muscles and draws the shoulder blades together.

Performed gradually it is very effective in releasing the entire shoulder girdle.

Work according to tolerance.

6 breaths should be ample.

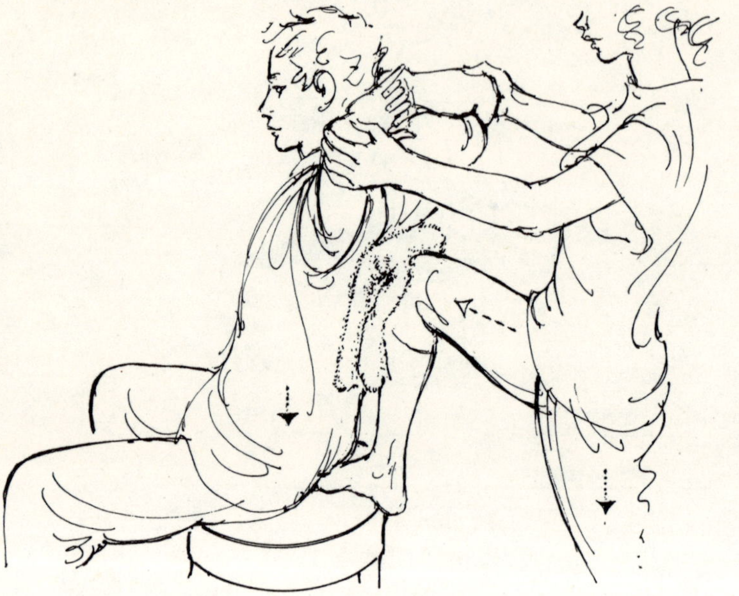

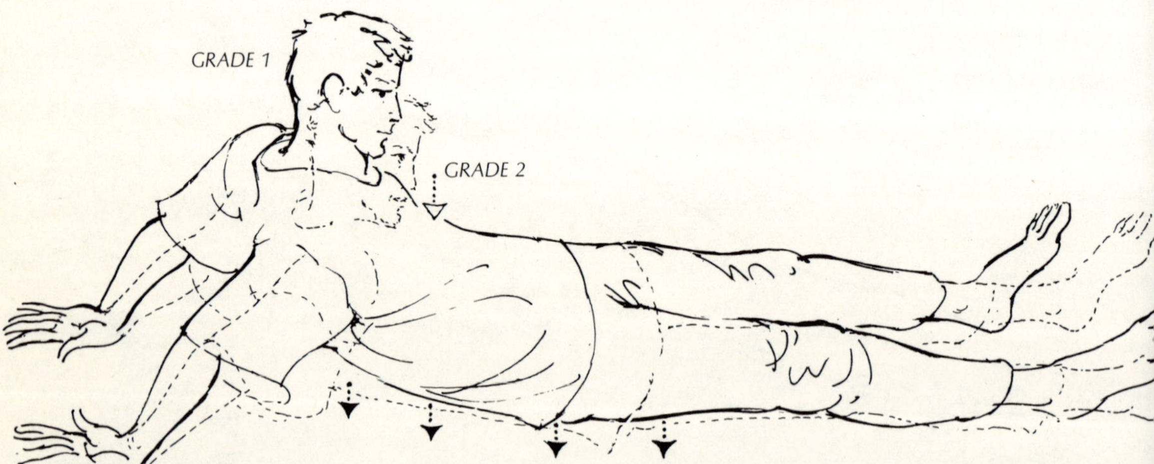

Shoulders 14

This technique exerts a strong pull at the front of the shoulder joint and of the upper arms.

Sit with your arms behind you at shoulder width and your palms face up.

Edge forwards leaving your hands fixed behind you until you feel the pull in the shoulders.

Each time you exhale allow yourself to feel heavy and your chest to sink.

Release for at least 6 breaths.

As the resistance in the shoulders dissolves, you can edge forward a little more to increase the pull.

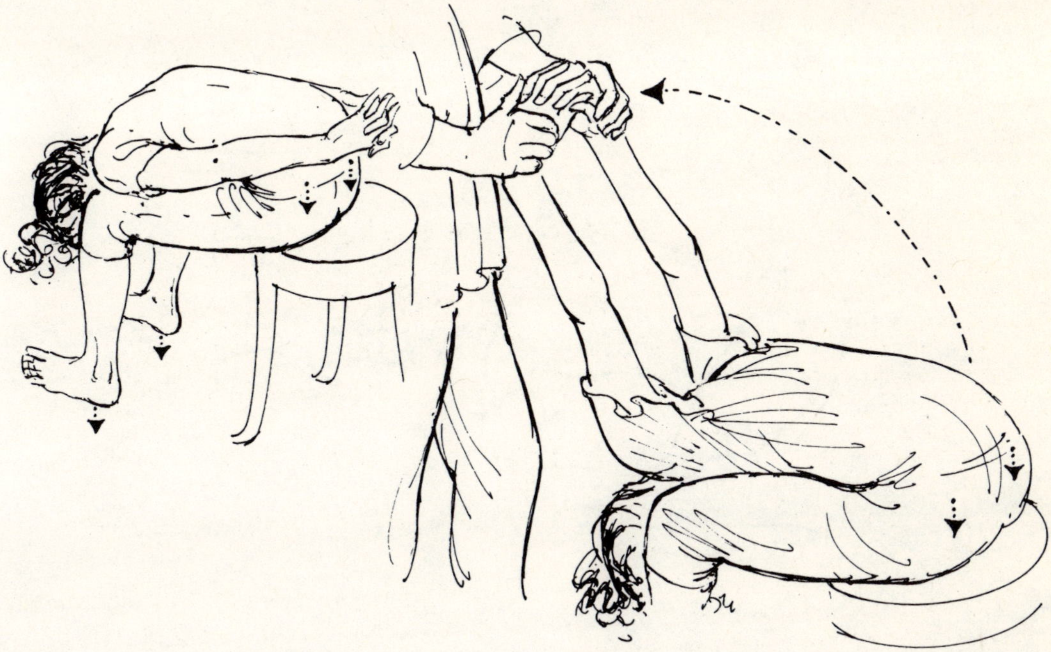

Shoulders 15

This assisted technique works on the same aspect of the shoulder girdle as the previous technique.

Sitting with your knees apart, feet flat on the floor, bend forward at the hips with your hands interlocked behind you.

Let your head drop and take a few breaths to release the shoulders.

The person helping holds your wrists and with a slight inward pressure to stop your fingers slipping apart gradually directs your arms upward and over your head.

Allow your chest to drop between your knees if you feel it is necessary.

Feel heavy in the pelvis and push your feet into the floor for stability.

If your shoulders are very stiff and your hands won't raise above the back of your pelvis for more than at least 30 cm this technique is not worth pursuing. Instead cultivate Shoulders 14 for a few weeks before trying this again.

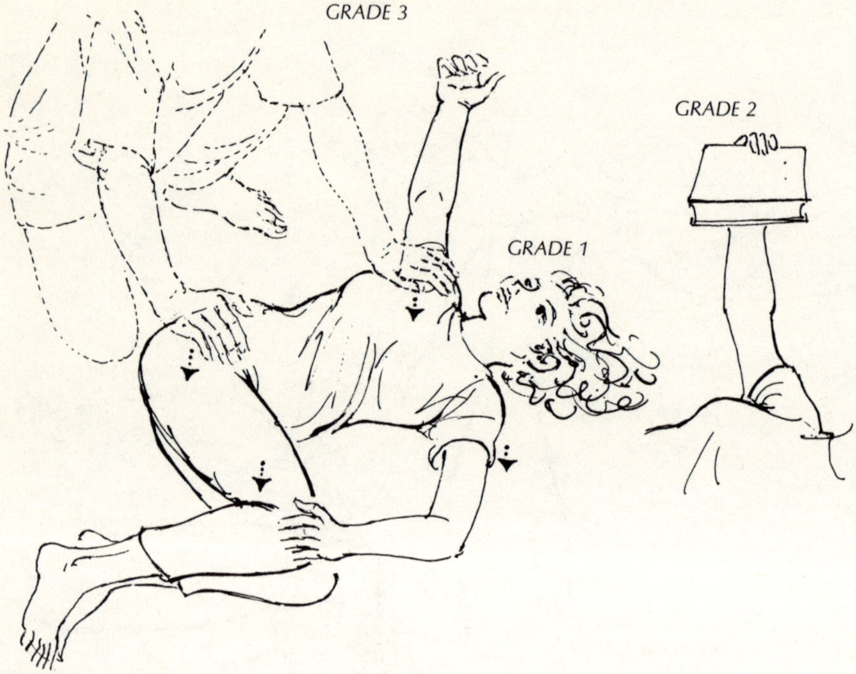

Shoulders 16

The common floor twist approached slightly differently can be used to localise movement at the shoulder joint.

Both knees are kept firmly together, taken down to the floor and held there with one hand.

The opposite arm is stretched out at a roughly 45° angle to the trunk.

Keeping the knees fixed drop the arm gently down towards the floor for at least 6 breaths, consciously releasing resistance in the armpit, the back of the shoulder or upper arm.

If necessary you can use a book or another person to exaggerate the technique.

Be inventive and try changing the angle of your arm to vary the location and intensity of the resistance.

You need to work through the angle of most resistance for the most benefit. With most people this angle lies somewhere between 30 cm and 10 cm from the ear lobe.

Work for enough exhalations to suit your tolerance.

Shoulders 17

If you have worked through a shoulder session, it is a good idea to get into the LRP with your arms outstretched and palms face up. Try to feel your shoulders from the inside using some basic breathing.

Each time you exhale imagine space inside your shoulders and weight through your elbows.

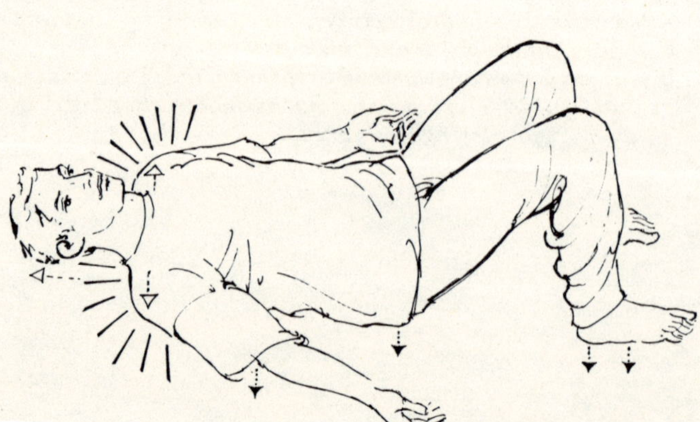

Elbows, Wrists and Hands

Those whose business it is to balance structure often consider the elbow, wrist and hand relatively insignificant in terms of total integration. But it would be incomplete to leave out any part of the structure, no matter how small its role in the overall mechanical function of the body.

Structural stiffness of the arms and hands is unlikely to affect the rest of the structure to any great extent. But many of the shocks and stresses to the arms and hands are absorbed through the shoulder girdle to the spine. Each upper extremity forms an entire unit, some muscles influence both the shoulder and the elbow and many muscles co-ordinate movement of the elbow, wrist and hand. Most arm and hand movements are initiated at the shoulders and progress through successive joints to the fingertips. Impediments to free flow often start at the shoulder and cause disharmony further down towards the hand. But finger, hand, wrist or elbow restrictions can transmit tension towards the shoulders and on a subtle level to the spine itself.

The elbows provide a stable link between the shoulders and hand and are unlikely to stiffen unless injured. But the wrists can stiffen insidiously and this may only show up when their full range of movement is tested. Long tendons from the forearms run through the wrists and are commonly prone to inflammation and pain. The fingers also tend to stiffen up considerably as we get older, they are rarely if ever stretched. Few people can bend their fingers backwards to form a right angle with their hand.

The freedom and balance of the elbows, wrists, hands and fingers may not have such a great part to play in the postures and movements of the body as a whole and they may not affect the rest of the unit to any great extent but there is no doubt that their freedom and balance effects the comfort, activities and general energy levels of each individual.

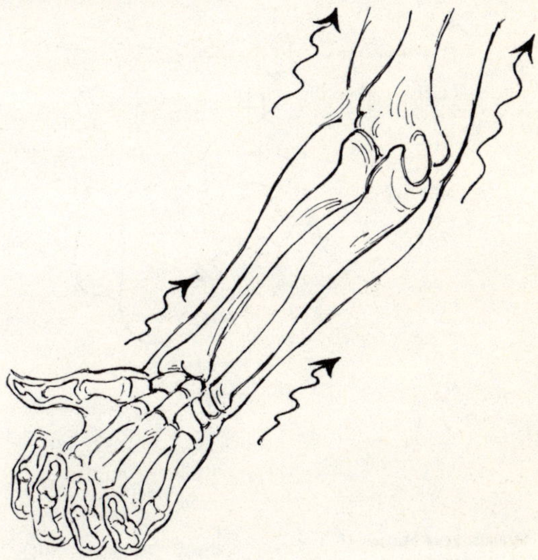

Wrist or elbow restrictions can transmit tension towards the shoulders and on a subtle level to the spine itself.

Stretching the Wrists and Hands

Wrists and Hands 1
Standing in the SRP imagine your hands as two heavy mittens filled with sand on two pieces of elastic.

As you exhale the weight of the mittens stretches and lengthens the elastic, the elastic of course being your wrists.

Visualise for enough breaths to perfect the imagery.

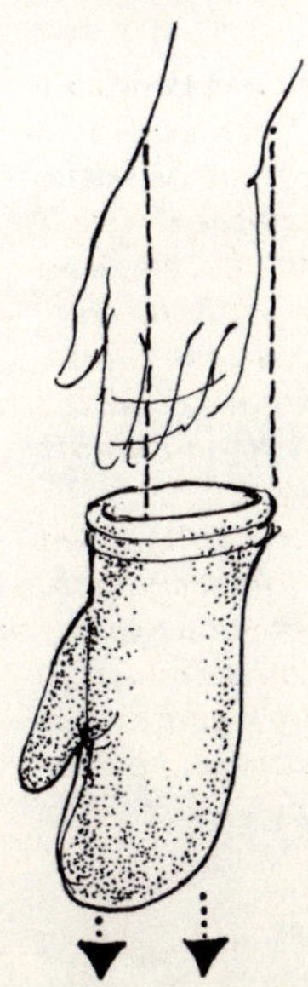

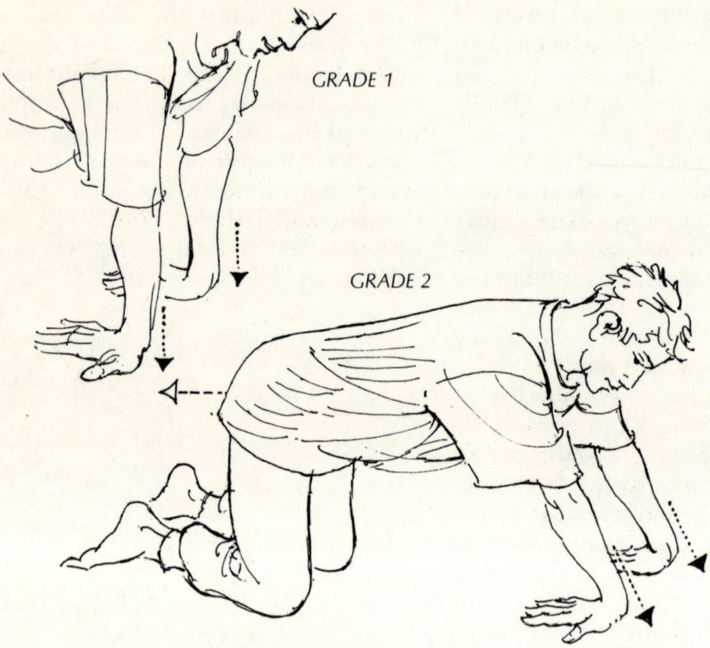

Wrists and Hands 2

Kneeling, put your palms flat on the floor with your fingers pointing towards you.
Your thumbs should be on the outsides of your hands.
Gently push the rims of your hands down as you exhale.
If this is easy, move your body backwards to increase extension at the wrists.
Work for 6 to 8 breaths.

Wrists and Hands 3

This technique uses the thumb as a lever to stretch the wrists the other way, e.g. use your left hand to stretch your right thumb in towards the front of your right forearm.

Eventually thumb and forearm touch.

Resistance is felt on the top of the wrist.

Work and release for at least 4 breaths on each wrist.

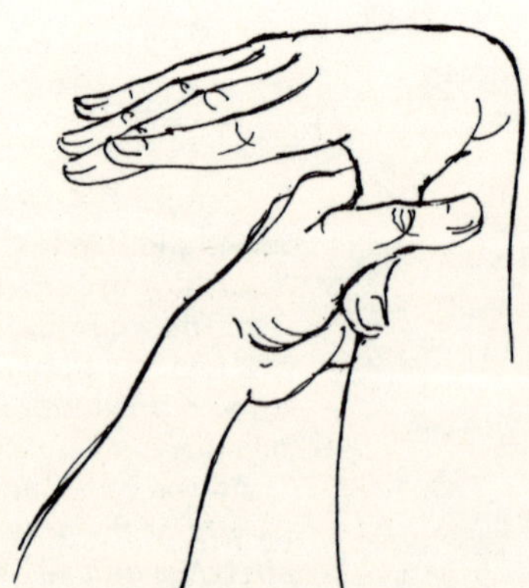

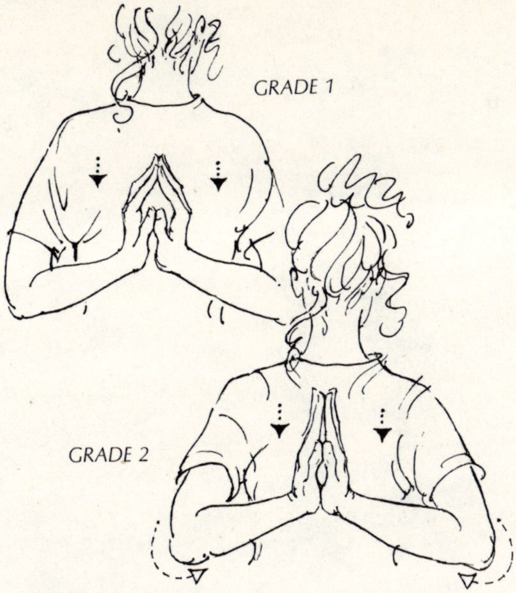

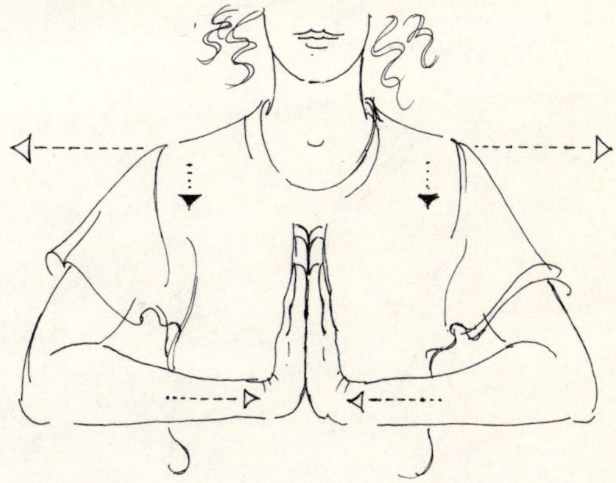

Wrists and Hands 4

Shoulders 5 can also be used for the wrists.
Hold and release for at least 6 to 8 breaths.

Wrists and Hands 5

This "prayer" position is good for the wrists.
Keep your shoulders down and broad.
Keep your hands a few centimetres from your chest and your forearms in line with each other and push the palms together for about 10 breaths.

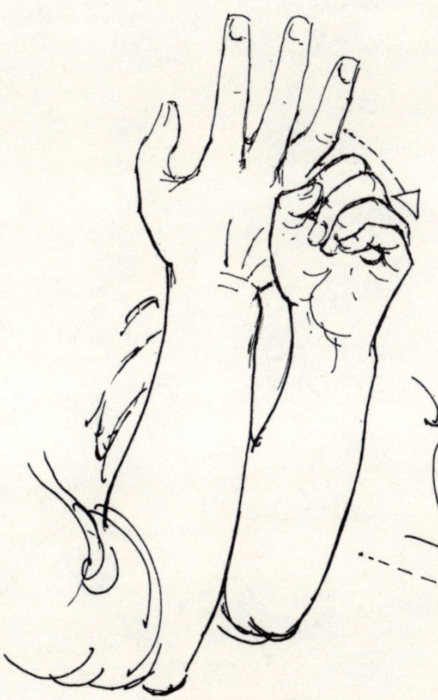

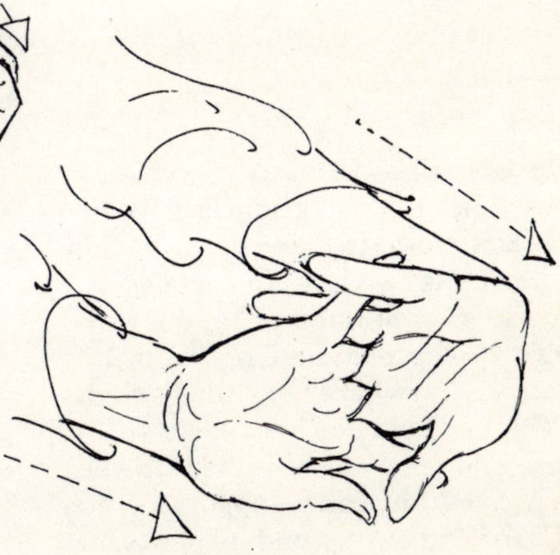

Wrists and Hands 6

Simply stretch each finger back until the resistance starts to "bite" and release for a few breaths.

OR

Interlock the fingers and stretch your palms away from you for a few breaths

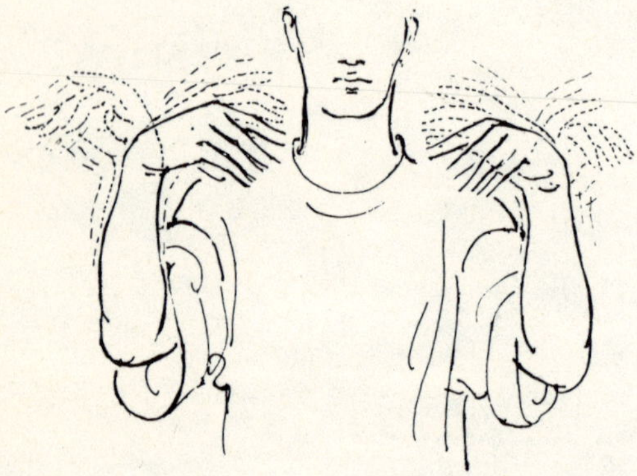

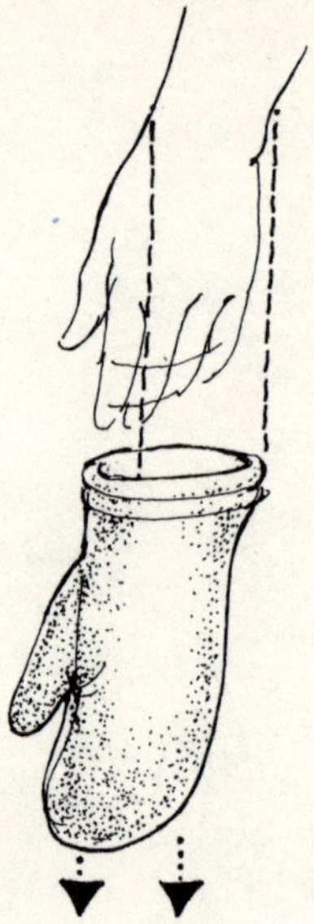

Wrists and Hands 7
To finish, loosely shake your wrists and hands and then stand in the SRP again and use the heavy mitten on the elastic technique (Wrists and Hands 1) to see whether the visualisation and the feel of the wrists have improved.

The Head

The position of the head and its movements on the neck both influence and are influenced by the structural freedom of the entire body. The head sits on the spine at a point just behind the joint of the jaw, in line with the entrance to the ear, and not as most people imagine somewhere near the back of the neck. The head weighs between 6 to 10 kilogrammes and acts as a top load on the spine, which gives it a secure support due to its natural opposing curves and its powerful muscles and ligaments. The head balances on the top vertebra, a small bony ring called the atlas. The atlas presents a very small surface on which the head can balance and the head and neck muscles need to be quite strong and in balance to move the weight of the skull efficiently. A head which is held habitually off centre inevitably stiffens the muscles of the neck and shoulders which

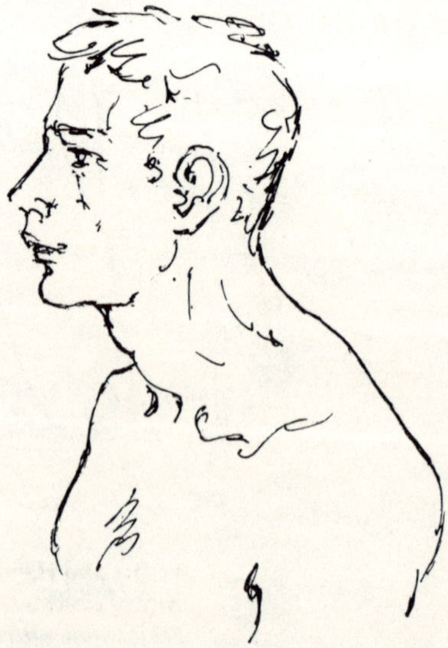

The most common fault is the head held too far forward.

help move and support it. The most common fault is the head being held too far forward to compensate for rigidities and imbalances further down. Often the joints between the atlas and the skull become jammed up on one side causing a sideways tilt of the head and habitual strain in the neck. Less common is the head that is held too far back: this usually co-exists with the spine that is too straight and poker-like.

When the head is off centre the neck is disturbed and the whole spine may be subject to strain, over-compressed in some areas and over-stretched in others. Conversely, when the structures below are rigid and off balance, the position of the head and its freedom on the neck and shoulders suffers. Head balance and freedom are most important: firstly, for local integrity of the neck—the less strain on the neck, the less strain on the vital nerves and vessels coursing through it that exchange fluids and information between the body and brain; and secondly for the integrity of the structure as a whole.

Centring the Head

Even though the overall structural work will ultimately centre the head, these few specific techniques for the neck will accelerate progress.

They are also valuable in de-stressing and decompressing this vulnerable upper region of the spine.

Head 1
Either standing in the SRP or sitting with a heavy pelvis and straight spine, visualise the crown of your head being lengthened upwards by a thin cord attached to a pulley on the ceiling.

Each time you exhale an imaginary figure pulls on the cord a little more.

This technique is extremely effective at freeing the neck from the shoulders and realigning the head.

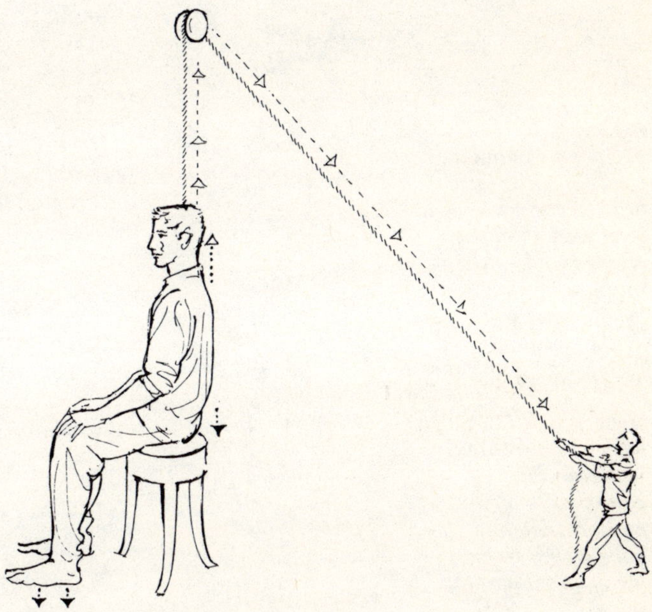

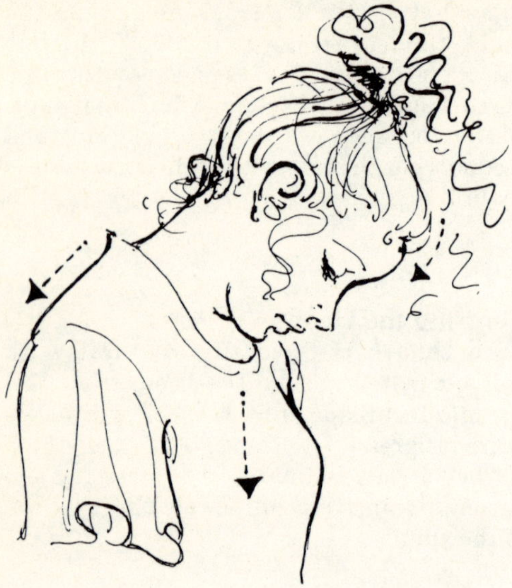

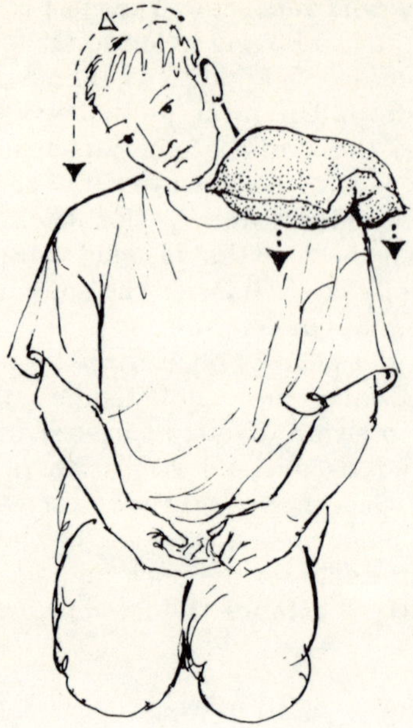

Head 2
Sitting or kneeling with your head bent, visualise the top of your breast bone sinking slowly down and inwards each time you exhale. Feel your head becoming heavier and the back of your neck and space between your shoulder blades releasing as you imagine your breast bone moving away from your chin.

Head 3
Sit or kneel with your hands on your lap and your elbows feeling heavy.

Drop your chin very slightly and softly side-bend your head to your right.

Close your eyes and imagine that someone has placed a heavy sand bag on your left shoulder.

Visualise clearly the texture and shape of the sand bag and sense it weighing down your left shoulder as your head and neck stretch and release to your right.

Only visualise and sense during your exhalations.

Practise for at least 6 breaths and then change sides.

Head 4
From your previous position with your head in the centre, keep your shoulders relaxed and softly rotate your head to look behind you.

Fix your eyes on a specific point on the wall, hold for a few seconds and then turn back to the front.

Repeat the movement and you will see that your eyes have moved beyond the original point on the wall.

Repeat gently 4 to 5 times and each time your eyes will focus on a spot even further than the original one.

Repeat the technique towards the other side.

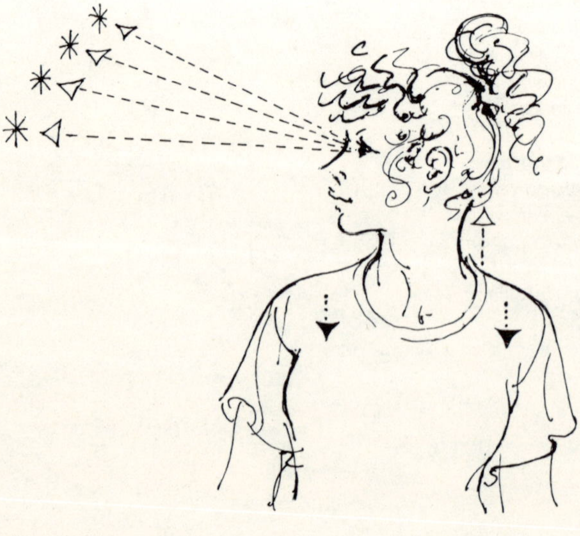

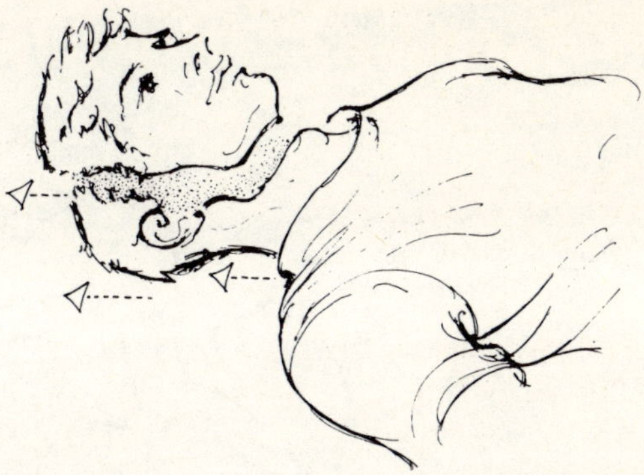

Head 5

From the LRP, with your hands out to the side, imagine your head as being in two halves, divided roughly into a front and back section where your ears are situated. Imagine that the back half has slipped downwards towards your shoulder blades.

Each time you exhale visualise this slipped back section slowly sliding upwards to realign itself with the upper section.

This technique provides a great sense of release at the back of the neck and upper part of the shoulders.

N.B. Use a folded blanket underneath your head if your neck is inclined to arch and your chin protrude upwards.

The Jaw

Most people have tension and tightness in the jaw which often relates to tension between the skull and the top of the spine. Few people know the exact location of the joint of the jaw but its movement can be easily felt by putting a finger directly in front of each ear and opening and closing the mouth. The jaw tends to protrude and move forward as it opens, and retract or move backwards as it closes. It can also deviate to one side which involves protrusion on one side and retraction on the other. The possible force in clenching the jaw has been estimated to be 242 kilogrammes. (This is demonstrated by the strong men who lift things between their teeth.) Tremendous tension can build up in the jaw and it can stiffen in a number of ways. It usually becomes restricted in opening fully, either on one side or both, and many people's jaws tend to deviate slightly to one side when they open their mouth wide. The three most chronic forms of jaw tension are reflected in the receding jaw, the protruding jaw and the clenched jaw which may exist in combination with the other two.

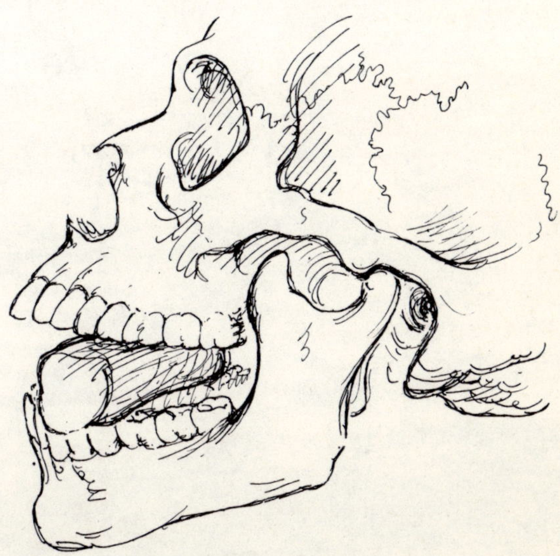

The possible force in clenching the jaw has been estimated at 242 kilos.

Releasing the Jaw

Jaw 1
Slowly run your thumbs from just in front of your ears, underneath your cheek bones to the corners of your mouth. Use enough pressure to feel the tissues stretching.

Keep the jaw loose and relaxed as you work. Repeat 4 or 5 times breathing slowly.

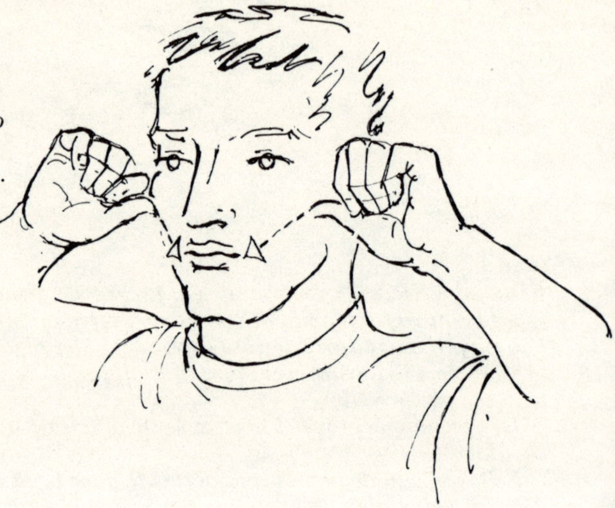

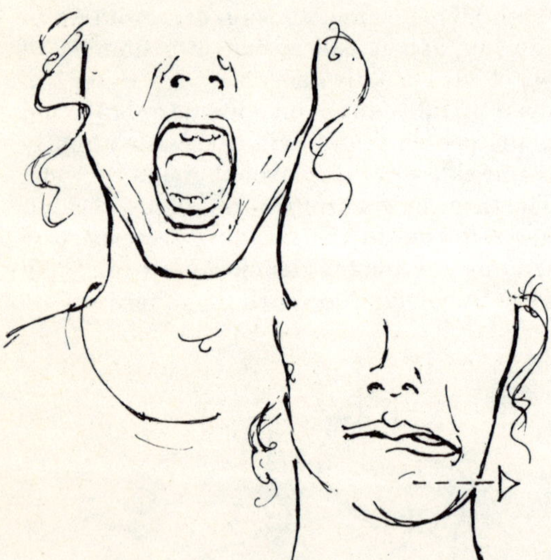

Jaw 2
Open your jaw as wide as possible without forcing and consciously release any sensations of tightness while breathing in and out through the nose for 4 or 5 breaths.

Then with your mouth slightly open and relaxed, gently deviate to each side, holding and releasing for a few breaths.

Structure and Cranial Fitness

THERE is a link between the structure of the body and the structure of the head and this can influence the health of the whole body. The head is a structure made up of 29 bones and the joints between them give the skull a slightly flexible and elastic quality. This quality allows the head to adapt to mechanical demands such as the absorption of shocks from physical trauma, changes of growth, and allowances for the subtle expansion and contractions that accompany emotional changes, breathing and other vital rhythms. Cranial osteopathy attaches great importance to the relationship between the cranial bones and the flexibility of the cranial joints, and deviations from a known normal pattern are used diagnostically and in treatment. Strains on cranial joints easily arise from trauma coming from outside the body e.g. accidents to the head or exaggerated pressures and stresses at birth. However, strains may also occur from compensations for restrictions in other parts of the body, especially the pelvis and the base of the spine. It has also been found that the ribs, the upper back and the legs may also be involved in cranial immobility and imbalance.

The first cranial bone to meet stress coming from below is the occipital bone, which forms the base of the skull and sits on top of the spine. It is the mediator, the link between the rest of the structure and the other cranial bones. Study of the cranial joints shows that when the body as a whole is off balance the occipital bone can get jammed or stuck either on one or on both sides against its neighbours, and this generally upsets the fine and subtle balance of cranial movement as a whole.

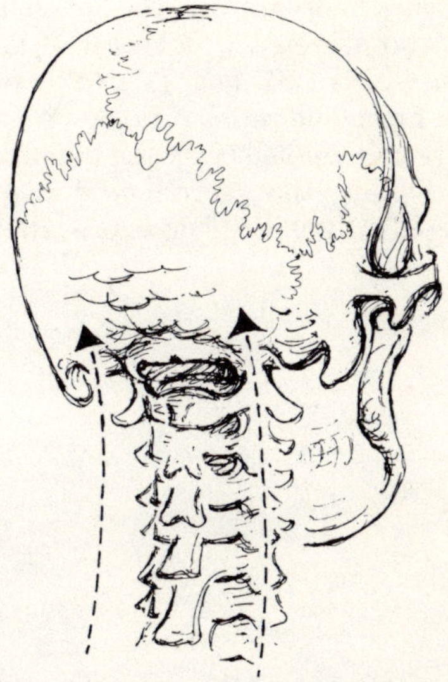

The occipital bone is the first bone to meet stress coming from below

As well as concerning itself with the effects of bony disturbances on hearing, vision, smell and other disorders local to the head, cranial osteopathy is also concerned with a series of distinct rhythmic impulses coming from inside the cranium. Scientific evidence suggests that these impulses relate to an inherent mobility of the central nervous system (brain and spinal cord), and the flow and fluctuation of a vital fluid, produced in the brain's cavities, called cerebrospinal fluid (CSF). Dr Andrew Taylor Still, the pioneer of osteopathy in the late 1800s, considered the CSF the most important element in the body and tried to influence its role in healing by treating his patients' heads as well as the whole body. A student of Still's, W. G. Sutherland, made further developments in this direction which led to the concept of cranial osteopathy.

The inherent mobility of the brain and spinal cord and the distribution of CSF is believed essential to overall health. CSF is thought to spread throughout the entire body, bathing all nervous tissue and aiding metabolism in general. CSF flow is largely controlled by the tension of a membrane in the head which extends down around the spinal cord as far as the sacrum. Cranial osteopaths enhance CSF flow by gently compressing the occipital bone. Such procedures have proved useful in improving arthritic disorders and are said to stimulate the immunity functions of the spleen, tone the liver and pancreas and stimulate the pituitary gland.

The cranial rhythmic impulse is known to cease temporarily when a person experiences fear, increase in the presence of oxygen and decrease as a result of fatigue. In other words CSF flow is stronger when you are fitter and more relaxed. When the structure as a whole is free and balanced the occipital bone, the sacrum and the membrane controlling CSF flow are all under minimum stress, allowing this nutritious fluid to circulate freely throughout the whole body.

Overall structural fitness is neither a replacement nor a substitute for the art and science of cranial osteopathy. There are a wide variety of imbalances that can occur between the skull's 29 bones from all kinds of accidents and birth traumas, many of which appear to be successfully corrected by skilled cranial therapists. But there is no doubt that improving structure overall reduces any cranial strains that can arise from below and the mechanism that distributes CSF is more likely to operate freely.

Structure and Health

THE media never tell us what percentage of the population is in good health. Disease makes the news, not health. We may learn that someone dies from heart disease every three minutes, or that cancer claims so many new victims each year, or that the demand for hip replacement surgery is on the increase. Disease-less people are not medical successes because health is automatic. It is taken for granted that most of us are born healthy and accepted that some of us will "get" diseases. Successes involve sick people being cured and disease is studied more than health because health presents no threat to life or the quality of life. But more and more people are realising that it may be more productive to have a science of health than a science of medicine. It must be more advantageous to study what *keeps* people healthy.

There are two ways of treating disease: fight it or prevent it. Orthodox medicine endeavours to kill the germ and cure the disease. Alternative medicine, however, as well as treating disease, concentrates on making the body healthy as an insurance against it. Many of us who are health-conscious make our own provisions against sickness and disease in the form of diet, exercise and so on. It is a fact that people who regularly work on their structure not only move better and have relatively few of the common aches and pains associated with getting older, but are also rarely if ever ill, or catch diseases.

Soil

Medical science has long regarded germs as the *cause* of many diseases. But certain pioneers in the germ theory of disease felt that it was the quality of the soil—the cells and tissues of the body—that was all important. They believed that the bacteria found in association with certain diseases was not the primary cause but the product of conditions in the body in which bacteria breed and multiply. Antoine Bechamp, who studied germs before Pasteur, wrote, "There are no germs and no bacteria which are intrinsically harmful in order to make men and animals ill, the primary cause of our diseases is always inside us." Naturopathy and traditional osteopathy have held this view for many years and believe that because most pathological cell conditions are fundamentally problems of deficient nerve, blood and lymph supply, poor soil is related to changes in this supply. Removing obstructions to this supply promotes health. Health resides in the cell, a minute replica of the entire person, which eats, drinks, grows, throws off waste matter and multiplies just like man. Healthy cell, healthy soil, healthy man.

The traditional bone-setters in European countries noticed that their treatments not only relieved strained and tired backs, but often were instrumental in aiding the recovery from disease. The spine has been used to treat the whole body, since long before there was any scientific explanation for this. All schools of structural therapy agree that health and disease are to some extent conditioned by structural health. The early osteopaths based their principles of disease on the fact that the human organism is self-regulating, health is automatic. Disease was merely a process during which health was struggling under difficulty and the treatment and prevention of disease simply involved the removal of obstructions. Structural fixations, particularly of the spine, were considered a major contributing factor to disease by creating a disturbance to nerve supply and fluid flow through the rest of the body. Structural adjustment was an essential factor in the approach to disease because adjusting bones, ligaments and muscles helped to decongest the circulation and free the nerves supplying all the cells of the body.

An unhampered organism possessed the machinery and qualities necessary for the prevention of disease. Removing structural ob(struct)ions helped to establish normal conditions in the body so that the healer and regulator within could do its work. Yoga has been saying this for thousands of years.

Good soil also depends on the immune system, made up of a vast army of cells which search out and destroy foreign cells, micro-organisms, bacterial poisons and tumour cells. It is well known that certain hormones secreted during stress suppress the immune system and decrease immunity. Psychological stress induces physiological stress, anxiety has its own biochemistry. Many people fall ill as a result of sustained periods of psycho-emotional stress. But we can deal with undue stress to a great extent by de-stressing structure. Releasing rigidity and tension increases physical and mental relaxation, and relaxation is the big de-stressor affecting both the hormonal and immune systems.

There is no doubt that the finer the structural adjustment of the body, the finer its fluid and nervous adjustment and the more effective its immune responses. The body can function best in resisting disease and maintaining its own health when it is structurally mobile and flexible. Freeing structure is not an attempt to cure disease but a provision to encourage health.

Suggested Combined Routines

Before starting any of these routines, read the general guidelines on pages 26–28.

Non-Graded Combined Routines

An 8-technique routine

Start in SRP
Ankles 7
Hips 2
Pelvis 2
Spine 4
Spine 9
Shoulders 10
Shoulders 11
Head 5
Finish in LRP

A 12-technique routine

Start in SRP
Feet 5
Feet 7
Ankles 4
Hips 8
Hips 9
Hips 15
Hips 22
Spine 4
Spine 11
Spine 13
Shoulders 16
Head 5
Finish in LRP

A 16-technique routine

Start in LRP
Ankles 12
Hips 8
Hips 9
Hips 20
Hips 24
Pelvis 5
Pelvis 6
Spine 5
Spine 15
Shoulders 6
Shoulders 11
Jaw 1 & 2
Head 1
Head 2
Head 3
Head 4
Finish in LRP

Low-Graded Combined Routines

An 8-technique routine

Start in SRP
Feet 4 Grades 1 & 2
Ankles 2 Grades 1 & 2
Knees 2 Grades 1, 2 & 3
Hips 11 Grade 1
Hips 12 Grade 1
Spine 7
Spine 17 Grade 1 or 2
Shoulders 7
Finish in LRP

A 12--technique routine

Start in SRP
Ankles 2
Ankles 3 Grades 1 & 2
Knees 3 Grades 1 & 2
Knees 10 Grades 1 & 2
Hips 3 Grades 2 & 3
Hips 26 Grade 1
Hips 21 Grade 1
Spine 14
Spine 16
Shoulders 4
Shoulders 5
Head 1
Finish in LRP

A 16-technique routine

Start in LRP
Hips 11
Hips 12
Ankles 7
Ankles 9 Grades 1 & 2
Knees 11
Knees 12
Hips 16 Grades 1 & 2
Hips 18 Grades 1 & 2
Hips 23 Grade 1
Hips 26 Grade 1
Spine 6 Grade 1
Spine 7 Grades 1 & 2
Shoulders 7
Spine 14
Spine 16
Spine 17 Grades 1 & 2
Finish in LRP

Some middle-grade combined routines

An 8-technique routine

Start in SRP
Ankles 3 Grades 2 & 3
Knees 2 Grades 2 & 3
Hips 17 Grade 2
Hips 19 Grades 1 & 2
Hips 28 Grades 2 & 3
Spine 16
Shoulders 14
Spine 18 B or C
Finish in LRP

A 12-technique routine

Start in LRP
Ankles 9 Grade 1 & 2
Knees 9 Grade 2 or 3
Knees 13 Grade 2 or 3
Knees 15 Grades 1 or 2
Hips 6 Grades 1 and 2
Hips 21 Grade 2
Hips 23 Grade 3
Spine 16
Spine 6 Grade 2
Shoulders 4 Grade 3
Shoulders 14
Spine 18
Finish in LRP

A 16-technique routine

Start in SRP
Spine 6 Grade 2
Hips 5
Knees 10 Grade 2
Knees 13 Grade 2 or 3
Knees 15
Knees 17 Grade 2
Hips 12 Grade 2
Hips 13 Grade 2
Hips 15 Grade 2
Hips 19 Grades 1 & 2
Hips 27 Grades 1 & 2
Hips 28 Grade 2 or 3
Spine 16
Spine 18
Shoulders 7
Shoulders 14
Finish in LRP

Advanced combined routines

An 8-technique routine

Ankles 8 Grade 4
Knees 2 Grade 4
Knees 7 Grade 5 or 6
Knees 10 Grade 3
Hips 11 Grade 3
Hips 27 Grade 2 or 3
Spine 17 Grade 3
Shoulders 7 Grade 3
Finish in LRP

A 12-technique routine

Start in SRP
Knees 2 Grade 4
Shoulders 4 Grade 3
Shoulders 14 Grade 2
Hips 26 Grade 2
Knees 13 Grade 3
Knees 16 Grades 1, 2 & 3
Hips 23 Grade 3
Hips 28 Grades 3 & 4
Spine 4
Spine 16
Spine 17 Grade 3
Spine 18
Finish in LRP

A 16-technique routine

Start in SRP
Feet 5
Ankles 9 Grade 4
Knees 7 Grades 5 & 6
Knees 14 Grade 2
Hips 11 Grade 3
Hips 12 Grade 2
Hips 6 Grade 3
Hips 19 Grades 2 & 3
Hips 27 Grade 2 or 3
Knees 10 Grade 3
Knees 5
Hips 28 Grades 3 & 4
Knees 16 Grade 1, 2 & 3
Spine 16
Shoulders 14 Grade 2
Wrist and Hands 2 Grade 2
Finish in LRP

A purely postural routine for everyone

SRP
Feet 1
Pelvis 1
Pelvis 2
OR
Pelvis 3
OR
Pelvis 4
Spine 1
Pelvis 6
Pelvis 5
Pelvis 7 Suitable grade
Pelvis 8

Some assisted routines

For the lower structure

Feet 9
Ankles 11
Knees 8
Knees 9
Hips 8
Hips 11
Knees 6

A hip session

Hips 8
Hips 9
Hips 10
Hips 11
Hips 12
Hips 20
Hips 30

A session for the Pelvis and Sacro-iliac Joints

SI 7
SI 2
SI 5
Pelvis 7
SI 8

A session for the Spine and Shoulders

Spine 12
Shoulders 8
Shoulders 13
Shoulders 15
Spine 15

A suggested 7-day routine piece by piece

Day 1: Feet and Ankles

Feet 1
Feet 2
Feet 5
Feet 6
Ankles 4
Ankles 7
Ankles 8
Ankles 16
Feet 11

Day 2: Knees

Knees 1
Knees 2
Knees 3
Knees 7
Knees 19
Knees 10
Knees 12
Knees 13
Knees 17
Knees 20

Day 3: Hips

Hips 1
Hips 2
Hips 3
Hips 4
Hips 6
Hips 10
Hips 11
Hips 12
Hips 13
Hips 15
Hips 17
Hips 18
Hips 24
Hips 31

Day 4: Pelvis

Pelvis 1
Pelvis 2
Pelvis 3
Pelvis 4
Pelvis 5
Pelvis 6
Pelvis 7
Pelvis 8

Day 5: Spine

Spine 1
Spine 4
Spine 6
Spine 8
Spine 9
Spine 11
Spine 14
Spine 15
Spine 16
Spine 17
Spine 18
Spine 19

Day 6: Shoulders

Shoulders 1
Shoulders 2
Shoulders 3
Shoulders 4
Shoulders 5
Shoulders 7
Shoulders 14
Shoulders 11
Shoulders 16
Shoulders 17

Day 7: Wrists, Hands, Jaw and Head

Wrists and Hands 1
Wrists and Hands 2
Wrists and Hands 3
Wrists and Hands 4
Wrists and Hands 5
Wrists and Hands 6
Wrists and Hands 7
Jaw 1
Jaw 2
Head 1
Head 2
Head 3
Head 4